AF859738

To G.B.G.

The Remarkable Rachel Romain

A novel by

James Gottesman

ISBN: 978-0-9911557-7-4 **JayEddy Publishing**

This is a work of fiction and all characters appearing in this work are fictitious. Any resemblance to real persons, living or dead, is purely coincidental. The actions of any real characters referred to in this novel are fictitious.

Factual events will be written in *ITALICS, although some facts of history are always debatable.*

ACKNOWLEDGMENTS

Thanks go to many. Gloria Brown Gottesman, my longtime co-conspirator, like always, she was brutally and painfully honest.

I need to thank the readers of the drafts, all friends, particularly, Chuck Caplan, Greg Gottesman, Don Gottesman, Susan Tapper, GBG, Gayle and Paul. If I forgot someone – oops.

Thanks to editor Sydney Weinberg, of London.

I always thank Diane Mackay Richie, the superlative editor for the Department of Surgery at UCLA and the first person to teach me how to write. She may not remember, but I do.

Although I listened to everything and everyone, I didn't always follow all their suggestions. Alas.

– JEG

Table of Contents

Merchant Ship – 1800s

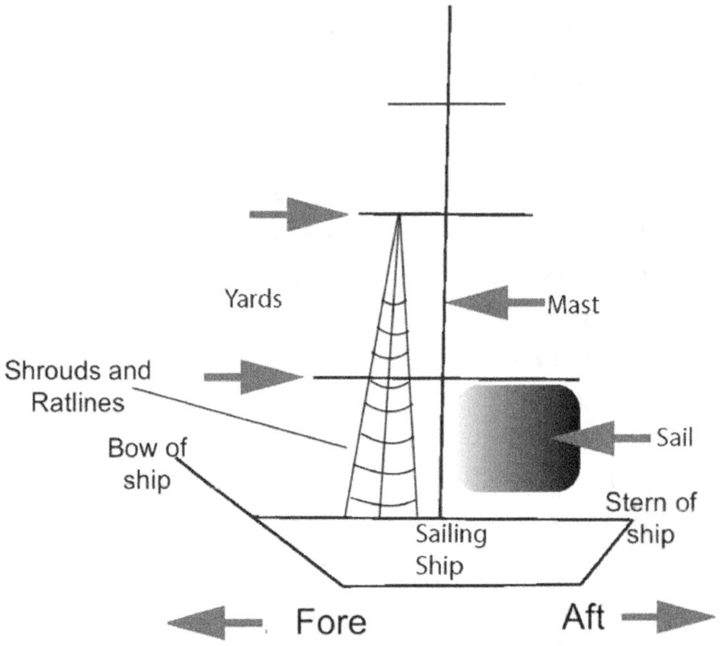

Yard: A long horizontal piece of wood attached to the mast and used to support and spread a sail.

Mainmast: Principal mast of a ship, usually the second mast of three on a sailing ship.

Shrouds: Ropes leading usually in pairs to give support to the masts.

Ratlines: small ropes fastened across a sailing ship's shrouds like the rungs of a ladder, used for climbing the rigging.

Racing Sloop 1860

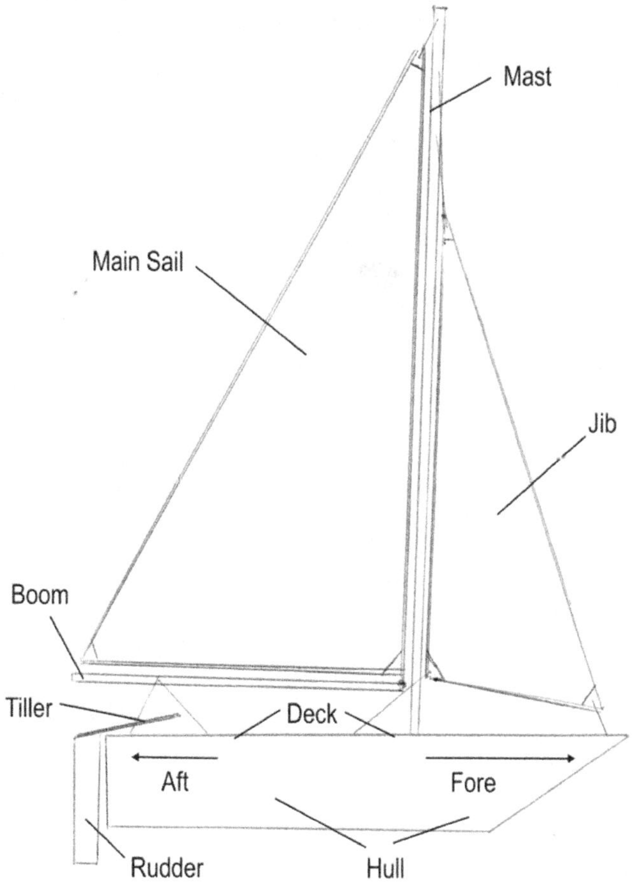

Isle of Wight and Southampton and the Solent

(southwest of London)

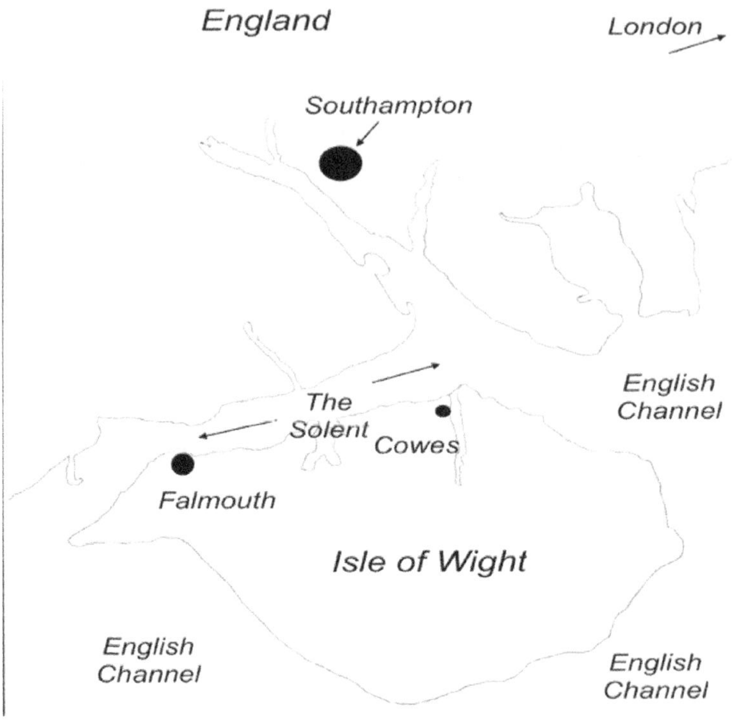

Battle of Chancellorsville, May 1, 1863 – First day
(Virginia, United States)

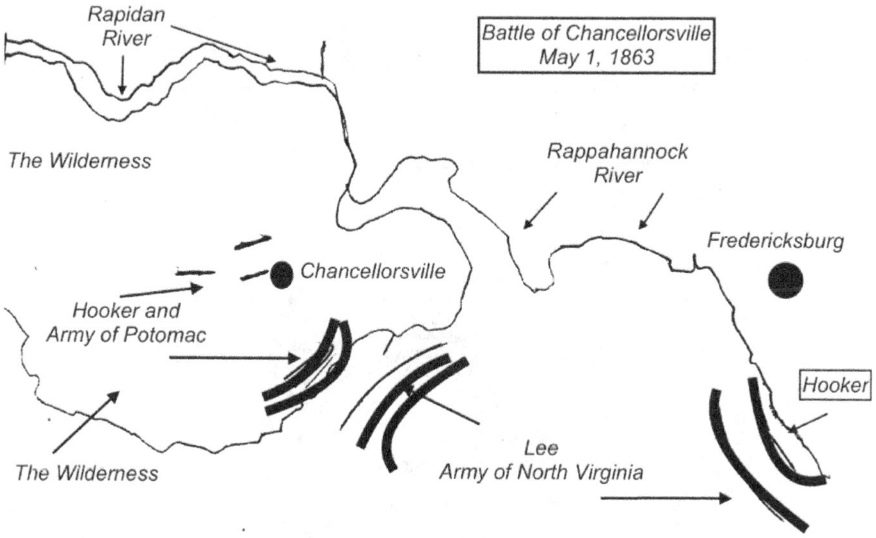

Battle of Gettysburg July 2, 1863 – Second day
(Pennsylvania, United States)

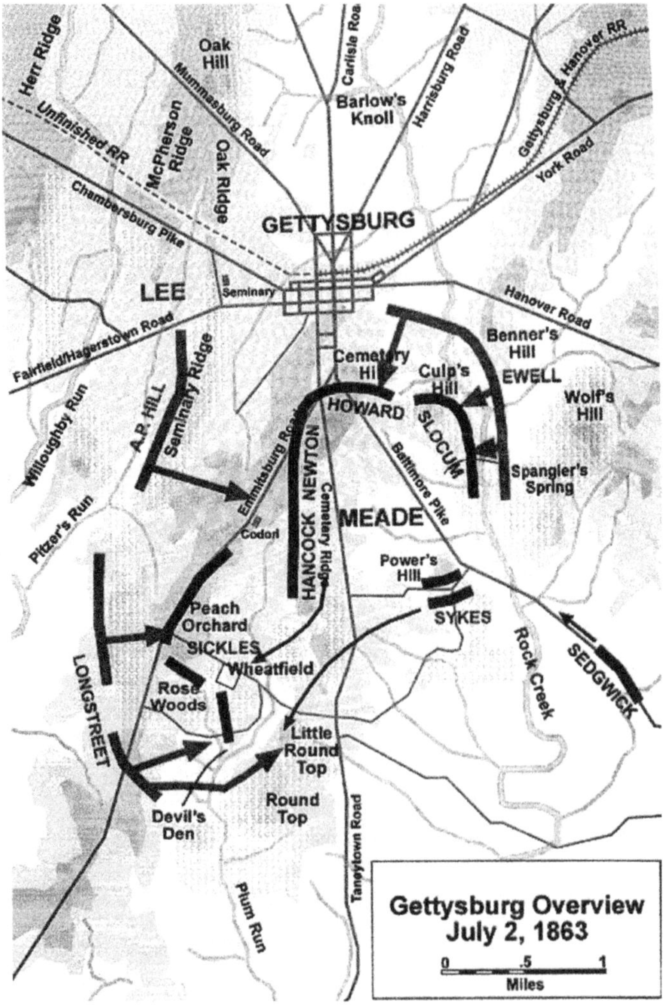

Prologue
December 1844 - East Indian Ocean
Ray/Rachel

The *Sol Quest*, a four-hundred-ton British merchant ship, had been fighting rain and gale winds for more than twelve hours. By sunset, the crew had reached the point of total exhaustion.

The ship's captain, Jacob Romain, rugged, with a weathered face belying his forty years, went below to check on two sailors injured trying to furl sails earlier in the storm. Romain left the helm in the hands of his trusted first mate, Ol' Tom Voz, a seasoned sailor, a decade older than his captain.

Fifteen minutes later, Ol' Tom came down to the sailor's quarters. "Cap'n, need you up top. We got a problem."

"Get it out, man," Jacob demanded, pulling on his oilskin topcoat.

Ol' Tom spoke quickly.

"The yard in the middle of the mainmast has cracked. I've sent a man up to release the sail but the yard won't hold his weight. I'm afeared the flapping sail will pull the entire mast down."

Arriving on deck, Jacob and Ol' Tom looked up to see the crack in the yard and the attached sail flapping hard in the wind. The mast itself was bent toward the weight of the dangling sail.

"We've got to get that sail released," Jacob yelled against the wind and rain.

Ol' Tom screamed back, "Anyone who climbs out on the yard will crack it the rest of the way. God help them then."

"Ray weighs less than fifty pounds and can do it."

"Too dangerous, Cap'n."

"We'll tie a safety line. At worst, Ray may dangle a bit but won't fall."

"Unless the entire mainmast comes down," Ol' Tom warned. "You can see it's stressed. Dunno know how much more it can handle before snapping."

"It needs to be done now. Once it's dark, we won't be able to free it. We've got to take the chance it won't snap whilst Ray's up there. We could lose the ship in this storm if we don't cut that sail loose," Jacob said.

Jacob left Ol' Tom to conscript Mick Backes, a strong sea dog, to climb the mast above the cracked yard with a safety line. Jacob ran down to his cabin to awaken Ray. The cabin boy was now ten years old, his only child.

Minutes later, Ol' Tom, Jacob and Ray stood on the windy deck looking up at the cracked yard.

"Ray, you think you can crawl out there and cut the sail loose?" Jacob yelled. "We've no other choices, or I wouldn't ask you."

"I'll give it my damn best, Cap'n," Ray yelled back. He always referred to Jacob as Cap'n, instead of father or Pa.

Despite the darkening sky, freezing wind and rain, Ray stripped down to a thin linen shirt and pants revealing a thin but wiry frame. Jacob tied the safety line at Ray's beltline, then Ol' Tom tucked his knife under Ray's belt. Mick, already on the mast above the cracked yard, held the other end of the safety line.

Without another word, Ray started up the ratlines to reach the cracked yard where it joined the mainmast.

Watching his only child climb toward danger, Jacob grabbed Ol' Tom's arm and muttered, "What have I done? God help me."

Ray looked up to see that Mick held the safety line tight, then crawled out onto the yard. A large crack in the yard opened and closed with each sway of the ship and each gust of wind. As Ray inched close to the crack, a huge wave tilted the ship to the port.

Jacob and Ol' Tom yelled, "Hold on," but it was too late. Ray was thrown over the side of the yard.

Jacob and the crew below let out a collective gasp as

Ray spun like a top in the wind, held up only by the safety line.

Mick pulled hard to allow Ray to grab the yard with one hand, stop spinning, and then get hold of the yard with both hands.

Ray swung a leg onto the yard, then Mick used the safety line to pull Ray back atop it. Undaunted, Ray waved to Jacob below, then inched over the crack out to the end of the yard.

Ol' Tom looked over to see Jacob's rigid face and said, "Cap'n. You might consider taking a breath here or there."

The yard's crack stayed open with Ray's weight, but did not break. Ray took Ol' Tom's knife and sawed through the line holding up the massive sail. The entire sail plummeted to the deck. Ray dropped the knife atop the released sail. As Ray inched backward toward the mast, the yard began to fail with a loud crack.

"Heave me up, damn you," Ray shrieked. "It's going."

Mick pulled tight, relieving all of the weight on the cracked yard until Ray reached the safety of the mainmast. Seconds later, the yard splintered with a cracking roar and separated, crashing to the deck, barely missing two sailors.

Ray and Mick descended the ratlines in double time. Teary-eyed, Jacob hugged and spun Ray in the air while Ol' Tom and the sailors on deck shouted, "Huzzah, Huzzah," congratulating Ray and Mick for saving the ship.

"You owe us an extra tot[1] of rum, Cap'n," Ray said with a smile, knowing there'd be no rum at all for the next ten years.

Mick nodded agreement. "Perhaps two tots, Cap'n."

After receiving a hug from Ol' Tom, Ray returned to Jacob's cabin to dry off and change clothes.

As Ol' Tom and Jacob watched Ray head off, Ol' Tom

---

[1] [1] Tot: about two and one-half ounces. The standard daily allotment of rum for sailors in the British Royal Navy.

put an arm around his captain's shoulder and said, "Got nerves of steel, that one. Remarkable."

Chapter One
London, December 1832 - twelve years earlier

Paul Romain, a successful Jewish merchant, traded in cotton, tea, and spices. Paul and his wife Gayle had a son, Jacob, early in their marriage.

Jacob took to the sea at sixteen with Paul's blessings, encouragement, and financing. By twenty-one, Jacob captained his own ship, *The Sol Quest.*

To the surprise and concern of everyone, Gayle became pregnant at the age of forty-two, twenty years after Jacob's birth. She delivered a healthy boy, Simon, but a postpartum hemorrhage took her life later that day.

Paul, devastated by Gayle's passing, never remarried, allowing nannies, tutors, and private boarding schools to raise Simon.

Simon, sixteen, returned home from boarding school for the winter holidays to find brother Jacob in town – a rare event.

Paul, now in his late sixties and used to being without family, shed his loneliness and appeared ebullient. Jacob, though broad-chested and powerful, was weather-beaten and seemed much older than Simon remembered from his last visit.

Being Friday night, Paul lit candles and standing together the three men chanted the Sabbath prayers before dinner.

"Tell me, little brother," Jacob asked, "are you ready to give up all this school nonsense and learn a real trade as I did at your age? I've talked to Father, and you'll join me next week as I sail to Venice, then Cape Town and back."

Simon had feared this offer. He looked despairingly at his father.

"I agree. Enough of schooling," Paul said. "It's time."

"No, Father. Please," Simon begged, shaking his head. "I've no desire to be cooped up on a ship."

Jacob's face darkened. It's an exceptional and lucrative life," he insisted. "After this voyage, I'll go mainly to the Far East. Ports of call and beautiful women everywhere. You'll love the excitement of Osaka, Singapore, Hong Kong, Bombay, Calcutta, Madagascar, and Cape Town. Once you're seaworthy, father will find you a ship of your own."

"That's right, son," Paul said. "It's time you joined the family business."

"No," Simon said with clenched fists, "I've heard you talk to father about life at sea the few times you've returned home. I've no desire to fight storms, loneliness, pirates or disease. I want to return to school to continue my studies."

"To what end?" Jacob demanded, exasperated.

"I want to be a physician, perhaps a surgeon. I like science and I'm good with my hands," Simon said. "I've known for a year. I didn't tell Father because—"

"Impossible," Paul cried. "You'd need to attend medical school and none exist in England for Jews."

"So I've been told by my professors," Simon said. "I would move to France, Prussia or Austria to study medicine."

Paul and Jacob exchanged a look.

"You don't know French or German," Jacob countered, shaking his head.

"I've finished my levels of Latin and *ich lerne Deutsh et j'étudie le français*. I'll be proficient in both in a year."

"Even if you succeed in getting a medical degree," Paul said at last, "The Royal College of Physicians and the College of Surgeons may not accept you. Even if they do, many of the hospitals won't allow you staff privileges."

"Jews are allowed now and with my education they cannot in good conscience refuse me," Simon said.

Paul and Jacob, surprised, looked at each other in silence as Simon seemed to have answers for all their concerns.

Jacob quipped, “A foolish decision, I fear, dear brother.”

“Enough of that, Jacob,” Paul said sharply.

Jacob looked surprised, but held his tongue.

Simon crossed his arms. “I’ve decided and I will not turn back. Even if I have to move to the Americas, I will be a doctor and surgeon.”

“Are you sure about this?” Paul asked.

“Yes. Absolutely.”

“Then I will support you,” Paul said. “You seem to have made up your mind anyway. I think your mother would have been proud. She wanted Jacob here in London to be a scholar, you know. She only reluctantly agreed to him going to sea.”

Simon smiled and gave his father a rare hug before sitting for dinner.

At the age of twenty-six, Simon finished his medical training in Strasbourg, France. On a fine spring day, he strolled to the post office to dispatch the last letter he’d send from abroad to his father:

1 March 1842

Dear Father,
I have passed my exams and will complete my studies this coming May. Then I will return home to begin my practice of medicine and surgery. Thank you again for your support and blessings. I am excited for the future.

During my training at the hospital, I’ve had the pleasure to make the acquaintance of a twenty-two-year-old Jewish-French nurse named Cynthie Goldhammer. She is widowed and childless and her English is excellent. Every week our affection for each other grows. I've asked her to marry me and she has accepted, although her family is not keen about her leaving France. Bowing to Cynthie's family's wishes, we will marry here in Strasbourg at the family's synagogue before returning home. I know you will adore her as I do.

Simon

Simon had cleared one major hurdle before sending the letter to his father – Cynthie's elderly parents. French Civil Code required parental permission for brides less than twenty-five years old.

The Goldhammers were ecstatic to have their youngest child find another spouse after Cynthie's first husband's tragic and untimely death. However, they had concerns about Simon being raised without a mother and his formative years spent in boarding schools away from his father.

When Simon sat with the Goldhammer's at their home to ask for her hand, he assuaged their fears. He explained that his father, Paul, had taught him life's important lessons - how to be a man and how not to be a father.

As a man, Simon would follow Paul's example - he would work hard, be honest, and attempt to earn the respect of the community. As a father, Simon would act in the opposite direction. Simon hoped that he and Cynthie would have a large family. More importantly, his children would stay home to be raised by Cynthie and himself. No child would be sent away to boarding schools.

Upon their arrival in London, Simon and Cynthie moved into Paul's large house with the hopes of starting a family. Simon opened an office and began his medical practice, with Cynthie acting as his nurse and assistant.

In time, Cynthie, tired of correcting English patients, began calling herself Cynthia.

With Simon and Cynthia as permanent residents of his house and London, Paul shed his loneliness. He adored Cynthia and when Simon was occupied, the father and daughter-in-law would spend hours together, reading, talking, playing card games and taking short walks.

A year into their new life, Paul died unexpectedly from an apparent stroke at the age of sixty-eight. Grief-stricken, Simon saw to his father's funeral the day after his death, per Jewish custom, and sat for the proscribed mourning period of seven days.

Jacob arrived in London a month later. Jacob and Simon had not seen each other for almost four years and Jacob had never met Cynthia. As expected, Jacob, the eldest, had power of attorney for all family matters. Jacob spent the first week at home assessing Paul's business and assets. Once accomplished, he called for a meeting with Simon without attorneys. Anxious to return to sea, Jacob, already wealthy, would not take advantage of his position. Simon demanded that Cynthia be present for any discussions.

Jacob, Simon and Cynthia sat in the family's parlor to hammer out the details of Paul's passing.

"I for one," Jacob said, "have no desire to stay in London and run Father's business."

"You don't have to ask me," Simon said. "I wouldn't know what to do."

"Agreed then, we sell the business and house and split the proceeds."

"No," Simon said, looking to Cynthia. "We would like to remain here in our house and start a family. I promise that whenever you return to London, you'll always have a welcoming place to stay."

Jacob assented, and the brothers shook on it. He boarded the *Sol Quest* two days later and set sail for Venice. He had no idea how his life would change and would not return to London for seventeen years.

Despite the various forms of antisemitism Simon faced by the London medical and surgical societies and hospital administrators, his medical practice flourished.

Simon, with Cynthia at his side, had a virtual monopoly on London's middle class Jewish population, which numbered thirty thousand. Only the wealthiest Jewish merchants, bankers and politicians used the prominent Gentile physicians who treated British royalty and members of the House of Lords.

When Simon applied for membership to the Royal College of Surgeons, his pedigree and medical diploma from Strasbourg left the College with no option but to accept him. Dr. Simon Romain reverted to Mr. Simon Romain in accordance with the uniquely British tradition of address for surgeons.[2]

In 1846, surgery made a monumental step out of the virtual obscurity with the successful introduction of general anesthesia (ether and chloroform). General anesthesia opened the doors to a variety of surgical procedures thought previously impossible.

Not surprisingly, Simon's surgical practice increased exponentially.

---

[2] *The uniquely British tradition of addressing surgeons as Mister dates well before the 19th century. Surgeons arose from the barber colleges – thus Mister rather than Doctor. The 'Mister' title remains to this day.*

Chapter Two
1848 – South China Sea
Rachel/Ray

Jacob Romain slept comfortably, gently swayed by the South China Sea. Rain clouds peeked through the damp shutters in his ornate captain's quarters and five bells[3] rang, meaning it was 6:30 a.m., and time to rise.

Just as Jacob opened his eyes, there came a knock on the door. This often meant trouble. When he saw that Ray's bunk was empty, he was alarmed at first, before remembering that Ray had asked for the 4 a.m. to 8 a.m. watch with Ol' Tom. He smiled as he opened the door to his cabin.

Ray, wearing an oilskin jacket, pointed hat and white linen pants, stood there with tears flowing down her cheeks.

"Cap'n," Ray wailed. "I'm dying."

"You're not," Jacob said, concerned nevertheless because Ray, now fourteen years old, never used histrionics to make a point. "What's the matter?"

"There's blood seeping down my leg. I could feel the wet but I thought it was rain. I didn't see it until Ol' Tom told me I was bleeding."

"C'mon in and we'll have a look," Jacob said, already suspecting the problem.

Jacob and Ray had shared the Captain's quarters since Ray became a cabin boy and permanent member of the *Sol Quest*'s crew at age six.

Jacob's wife, Ray's mother, had died when Ray, born Rachel, was one. Rachel, raised by nannies in Hong Kong, saw her father seldom, ached for his attention and threw tantrums whenever he sailed away. Years earlier,

---

[3] Bells: Ship's bell time originated in sailing ship days, when the crew on duty four hours, then off four hours. One stroke of the ship's bell indicates the first half hour of the watch. Then an additional bell is struck for each succeeding half hour. Watches began at 0400, 0800, 1200, 1600, 2000 and 2400.

when Paul Romain sent young Simon to boarding school, Jacob had argued that Simon should be kept at home. Jacob's plaints fell on deaf ears.

Jacob then had the same predicament with his motherless daughter and decided to bring her on board the *Sol Quest.* Jacob knew there were no female sailors, and he needed to raise Ray, Rachel's new name, as a boy and keep her real gender a secret. Other than Ol' Tom, Jacob believed that no one on the *Sol Quest* knew that Ray was a girl.

Jacob had explained long ago the differences between male and female anatomy to Ray, but hadn't described menstrual cycles. But now Ray's body was changing. There was a sinking feeling in Jacob's gut; the ruse couldn't last forever. They would need a new plan.

"Have a seat," Jacob said resignedly as he went to his sea chest and removed the menstrual cloths he'd secretly purchased in Hong Kong a year earlier. He spent the next hour explaining, as best he could, the changes that puberty would bring.

"It's Friday," Jacob said, "I'll be back in a couple of hours and give you some time to think. Tonight, we can light the Sabbath candles together. Okay?"

Ray could only nod acceptance.

Jacob needed advice and headed out of his quarters to look for Ol' Tom.

"Figure we're 'bout four days from Singapore if the winds hold," Ol' Tom said when Jacob joined him on deck.

"S'pose so," Jacob responded.

"You got a problem on your hands," Ol' Tom said.

"You asking or telling?"

"Telling. Ray's about to be grown and cropped hair won't hide it no more. The crew's been suspicious ever since her shirt got drenched in that sun shower outside Hong Kong. And she gets prettier by the day. They'll give her a wide berth as long as they be sober, which ain't too often. I'd be worried and she's gotta be prepared."

"Ray sleeps in my cabin," Jacob said. "She's quick, strong, and carries a folding dirk[4] with a Marlin spike."

"Little that'll do if she's surprised. You can't be letting Ray go ashore with the men alone no more. If they get soused, you don't know what they might do and they may not be able to protect her from others."

"I'll talk to the men."

Ol' Tom shook his head. "Cap'n, you're not listening. I'd give it six months, a year at most. The *Sol Quest* will be no place for her."

"She won't take kindly to being put ashore," Jacob lamented.

Ol' Tom nodded agreement. "I'd rather face a typhoon in a bathtub than have that conversation."

---

[4] Dirk: a long straight-bladed dagger favored by naval officers

Chapter Three
Simon and Jacob
London – 1849

While Simon became a successful surgeon with Cynthia at his side, the couple had no success having a child. Cynthia became pregnant soon enough after arriving in London, but one miscarriage after another followed. The large house they inhabited remained empty, save for themselves and a Scottish housekeeper. Even Jacob, promised a bed whenever he visited London, had not returned since Paul's death.

At thirty-nine-years old, Cynthia was four months into her seventh pregnancy and confined to bed by her obstetrician. Simon, sitting in his parlor reading a medical journal, heard screams from their upstairs bedroom.

"No. No. No. No."

Simon knew what the screaming meant. He ran to their darkened bedroom to find Cynthia on her side weeping. Jacob lit a candle, approached their bed and found the bedsheets soaked in blood.

"Oh, my poor dear wife," he said. Sitting on the edge of the bed, he kissed her sweaty forehead and stroked her hair until she calmed.

"I've disappointed you again," Cynthia wailed. "Will you forgive me?"

"You could never disappoint me," Simon said. "I love you and that is all I'll ever need."

After Simon changed the sheets and helped Cynthia into a fresh nightgown, he sat on the side of the bed holding her hand. Aided by a dose of laudanum, a mixture of opioids and high-proof alcohol, Cynthia closed her eyes and found sleep. Simon, still dressed, laid next to her with his arm over her shoulder and wept. A thought swirled in his head; his deceased parents would have no grandchildren to carry on the Romain name because he believed with certainty that

Jacob had shown no intention of ever marrying or having children.

...

Another year passed. Cynthia had not become pregnant, nor would she again.

Simon and Cynthia were preparing to leave for a friend's house to celebrate a birthday. They'd almost finished dressing when a loud knock sounded on the house's front door, audible even in the upstairs bedroom.

A moment later, the Romains' housekeeper, Sharron MacRosie, appeared outside the open bedroom door. Sharron, a red-haired, blue-eyed, widowed Scottish woman in her mid-forties from a village outside Glasgow had been working in the house for more than a decade,

"Ma'am," Sharron said.

Cynthia asked, "Is there a message?"

"Nae, Ma'am, it's a weathered man who says he's the doctor's brother, a Mr. Jacob. I had no idea who he might be. But he bears a resemblance to the doctor."

Cynthia shook her head at the surprise visit. "How wonderful, but what a time to have this happen. We've not seen Jacob in more than seventeen years. Did you let him in? He'll stay in the guest room and you'll need to ask if he's hungry."

Cynthia turned to Simon, who was exiting his closet. "Your brother dropped out of the heavens and is standing in the doorway."

"Nae, Mr. Jacob didn't come in," Sharron said. "He went back to the street and I watched him pull a bonnie wee lad out of the carriage who dinnae want to come. I left the door open and ran to tell you."

"A boy?" Simon asked. "Are you sure?"

"Yes. I know a lad when I see one."

"Of course. We know you do," Cynthia said.

"Skinny but wiry. Wouldn't wanna tussle with him.

Short hair and dressed like a sailor," Sharron said with hands on her hips. "I'm guessing 'bout fourteen, but that's a guess. Mr. Jacob was dragging the lad by the collar toward the front door."

"He dragged him?" Simon asked.

"The lad dinnae wanna come, howling the whole way with bad words I cannae repeat. I thought the lad a ragged beggar in need of a scrubbing and a bar of soap in his mouth," Sharron added.

"Oh, my. Were their others?" Cynthia asked.

"Saw no one else, Ma'am."

Cynthia turned to Simon. "We need to go down and see what trouble your brother brings. I'm afraid we'll miss the party." Addressing Sharron, she added, "Put Mr. Jacob in the parlor and offer him any refreshment he desires. See if Mr. Jacob will let you take the boy downstairs and bathe him. Burn the lad's clothing if you think he carries lice."

Sharron had already taken the ragamuffin down to her quarters to commence the much-needed bath when Simon and Cynthia entered the parlor to meet with Jacob.

Jacob, sitting in a Victorian parlor chair and nursing a self-poured double shot of Scotch, put the drink down and stood.

"It's been too long," Simon said, embracing his brother. "We're happy to have you home. Tell us who've you brought with you."

"It's a bit of tale," Jacob said.

"Sit down, please," Simon said, gesturing to the same chair as he and Cynthia settled on the sofa opposite. "We had an engagement tonight, but we'll send our housekeeper to the Goldman house with our regrets. Please, tell the whole story."

"After leaving Britain in the fall of '40," Jacob began, "I sailed directly to Venice to unload finished cotton goods for Thomas Knapp and Sons. My intent was to sail immediately for Cape Town, but during the last days of the voyage to Venice, the *Sol Quest's* hold began to leak. This forced me to bring her to a Venetian dry dock. That delayed my leaving for three months. I had no choice but to remain in Venice, where I lost most of my crew."

"Go on," Cynthia said cajolingly. "You've told us nothing!"

"Knowing I'd be there for a while, I went shopping for a dinner suit. As I perused the finest Venetian wools in a tailor shop near the Ghetto Novo[5], a Jewish gentleman entered to look for a suit as well. He was accompanied by his daughter, Ricca.

As I turned to greet them, the tailor must have heard me gasp. Ricca had piercing violet eyes, a silk-like complexion, and curly auburn hair. It was as if time stood still for the longest moment. Anyway, having no friends in Venice and cognizant of our shared heritage, I befriended the gentleman and we joined together in selecting material. In the end, Ricca chose for both of us. Ricca's father, Marco Cordova, a banker to the Doges, invited me to his house that evening for dinner."

"You said yes because of the daughter?" Cynthia interjected.

"Of course. I'm human," Jacob laughed. "After dinner, I asked permission to call on Ricca the next day, and the next and the next."

"I can see where this is going," Simon said with a smile.

"You'd be wrong," Jacob replied. "I had no desire to become a banker or a landlubber and I let that be known. I love the freedom and adventure on the open seas. When Mr. Cordova realized I wouldn't stay in Venice, he and Ricca's mother decided they would not

---

[5] Ghetto Novo: a small, fortified island in Venice, formerly a foundry, where the Jews were forced to reside from 1516. Ghetto Novo was the first ghetto in Europe and connected to the city by two gates. The origin of the word '*ghetto*' come from the Italian word for *foundry*.

let her marry a vagabond who would be gone most of the time. They demanded I cease my visitations."

"So then what? He changed his mind?" Cynthia asked.

"No. Mr. Cordova remained steadfast that I would never be his son-in-law and refused me all contact with Ricca."

"Please, Jacob," Simon said, "get to the point!"

"Ricca, on the other hand, was spirited and outspoken and yearned for adventure. She had never been more than ten miles outside of Venice and felt cloistered like a nun. On our walks and gondola rides through Venetian canals, I told her of Arabia, Cape Town, Bombay, Singapore, Shanghai and Osaka. She wept at the thought that she might never see them in her lifetime."

"I see a fight brewing between daughter and father," Cynthia said.

"Exactly. She told her father she was in love and wanted to go with me. Not surprisingly, he locked her in their house and sent a message to me that if I came anywhere near his home, he'd have the Carabinieri arrest me."

"Who are the Carabinieri?" Simon asked.

"Some form of national police. All a bit untethered."

"So what happened to you and Ricca?" Cynthia asked. "You're killing me."

"I didn't see Ricca again and believed I never would. Six weeks later the *Sol Quest* was ready to sail with a watertight hull and a new crew," Jacob continued. "I then received a message, supposedly signed by Mr. Cordova, that, as a token of friendship and forgiveness, he would send a trunk of fine local wines to the dock on the day of my departure."

Simon laughed. "You were certain it wasn't gunpowder in the trunk?"

"I hadn't thought of that at the time. Perhaps I should have," Jacob said, grinning.

"Most definitely should have," Cynthia interjected.

"Let me finish. On the flood tide, an hour before sailing the following morning, a heavy, padlocked trunk arrived as promised. The delivery men told me to be careful as the wines were loosely packed. I had it gently handled and stowed in my cabin."

"What in God's creation does this have to do with a young boy," Simon said.

"Let me finish, blast it," Jacob said. "After we pulled away from port, Mr. Cordova and a handful of Carabinieri appeared on the dock frantically waving their hands. Thinking Mr. Cordova was wishing me well, I bowed and waved back. I understood later that he wished me dead."

"I'm confused," Cynthia said. "Could Ricca have been pregnant?"

"No," Jacob smiled.

"I'm so confused," Simon said.

"But when we cleared Venice past the Punta Sabbioni out into the Adriatic, I left the helm with my First Mate and headed to my quarters. To my surprise, I found the trunk pried open from the hinges."

"Was the wine gone?" Cynthia asked.

"There was never wine," Jacob said with a broad smile. "There was only Ricca. She had forged the note, slipped out of the house, and paid two men to deliver her in the trunk to the ship."

Simon and Cynthia's eyes and mouths opened to their fullest.

"You must be joking," Cynthia said. "What a tale."

"Not a tale. We were married by a rabbi in Casablanca three weeks after leaving Venice. Ten months later, in Singapore, our daughter Rachel was born. She was named after both our grandmothers. But I call her Ray."

"A strange nickname for a girl. Where are Rachel and Ricca now?" Simon asked.

"Ray's being bathed by your maid," Jacob said.

"I'm confused," Cynthia said. "Our housekeeper told us the child was a boy."

"No. Ray's a girl, actually a young woman of sixteen. And that's the issue," Jacob said.

"This is all odd. When do we get to meet Ricca?" Simon asked.

"Never, sadly," Jacob said, bowing his head. "She passed."

Cynthia gasped. "Oh, my. What an awful turn of events. May her memory be for a blessing."

Tears formed in Jacob's eyes. He removed a cloth from his pocket, wiped the tears and said, "Thank you for the thought. Her memory will always be a blessing."

"Go on, my dear brother." Simon said. "There is more to the story."

"Ricca got her wish to see all the ports I had told her of. She loved the ship and I was as happy as a man can be. She got pregnant again soon enough after Ray. The baby, a boy, was born at sea, months early, a few days from Cape Town. The baby died that day. Ricca died two weeks later in Cape Town of childbed fever."

Cynthia said, "I'm so sorry."

"But you had a one-year-old daughter to care for," Simon said. "Why didn't you come home, or return the child to the grandparents in Venice?"

"I didn't dare go to Venice and face the wrath of the Cordovas. They would have blamed me for kidnapping and their daughter's death. I had heard through passing ships that if I ever strayed near Venice, they'd have me drawn and quartered. I didn't want to return to London because I wouldn't have stayed, and who would have raised Ray? I couldn't do to Ray what father did to you and send her away to be raised."

"What did you do?" Simon asked.

"I found a widow in Cape Town whose children had left home. She had been a caretaker for an elderly merchant who had recently died. She came on board and we sailed back to Hong Kong. I made only short runs from that point until Ray turned six. Ray was unhappy and wanted only to be with me. I transported the widow back to Cape Town with a generous stipend. Ray has been on board with me for the past ten years."

"Your ship was no place for a young girl," Cynthia chastised him.

"I didn't see it then. I kept Ray's hair short and raised her as a boy. I called her Ray, rather than Rachel, and that's how everyone knew her. Only my first mate, Ol' Tom, knew the truth of it. Ray loved the ship and the seamen treated her as a cabin boy."

"So, what now?" Simon asked.

"Ray's turning into a woman in every way. Sailors, on my ship or in port, cannot be trusted, particularly once three sheets to the wind. We've already had some issues and one close call after another. One on the ship and a few in ports. I fear for her safety. I've had to padlock Ray in my quarters more often than you need to know."

"Are you here to stay, my brother?" Simon asked.

"Not if I can help it," Jacob said. "I'm a sea captain and dreaded the life I might have spent in Venice. I need to be at sea."

"Ray ... uh, *Rachel*, can't be on a ship anymore. What are you thinking?" Cynthia asked.

"I want her to be around family, not in a boarding school like Simon. As I said, I had fought with father believing Simon should have remained home," Jacob said, with a sniffle and a shake of his head. "I'm here to plead with you to raise her here in London. Teach her to be a woman. Please."

Simon and Cynthia reeled backward as if kicked by horse. Unprepared for Jacob's plea, they looked at each other and then back to Jacob.

Jacob, believing the response of his brother and sister-in-law to be negative, sat up and steeled his jaw. "Our arrangement on settling father's estate and for you to keep this house was a promise of a bed and room whenever I came to London. Why would that not be true of my child?"

"Goodness, Jacob," Cynthia said. "Who do you think we are? Of course we'll take her."

Jacob's shoulder's relaxed as the weight was removed from his chest.

"Yes. It would be our honor to care for her," Simon echoed Cynthia's declaration.

"Thank you but it won't be easy," Jacob continued. "Ray wasn't raised to be a lady and she knows none of the societal norms or rules that she would have learned if raised in a fine London home. She's smart as can be, but headstrong and impulsive. If a sailor or anyone trusts her straightaway, she loves them in an instant. If they don't trust her, she'll never like them. She thinks and talks like a sailor, and swears like one too. She can repair a torn sail on the topmast in a gale and is stronger and more agile than half my ill-gotten crew."

Simon shook his head, having no idea what to say.

Jacob added, "I promise I'll be back every couple of years to visit. Please. Give it a try and if it's truly impossible, then you can place her in a boarding school."

Cynthia said, "We'll figure it out. You mustn't worry."

Sharron entered the room followed by Rachel, now bathed, wrapped in towels, and wearing a clean high-collared nightshirt of Cynthia's. Her angry violet eyes and short, wet, reddish hair lit up the room. Sharron, hands on her hips, announced, "This is nae a young lad. It's a bonnie lass but as strong as a longshoreman."

"We know. We've just heard her tale," Cynthia said as she stood to approach Rachel.

Sharron added, "If I didn't know better, with her hair color and eyes, she'd fit in with half my village outside Glasgow. Dirty mouth and all."

Jacob laughed. "She's a wonder and looks like her mother. Ol' Tom and I decided her hair had to be kept short when we brought her on board. When she lets it grow, there'll be curly locks like Ricca."

"No wonder you fell in love," Cynthia said as she took both of Rachel's hands in hers. "I'm your Aunt Cynthia, Rachel. Welcome to London."

Rachel shook her head violently and freed her hands. "I'm not Rachel. That's not my name."

"It is your name. Is it not?" Cynthia asked, her gaze moving uncertainly between Jacob and Rachel.

"So father says, Ma'am. But my name's Ray. May God damn anyone who calls me another."

Cynthia, stunned by the coarse language, took a step back.

"That's enough out of you, sailor," Jacob barked at his daughter. "Watch your mouth."

Rachel spun to face her father and tugged on the nightshirt. "Cap'n. I feel like I've been lashed to the mainmast in this. I can't be here. I need to get back to the *Sol Quest.*"

"She calls you Captain?" Simon asked.

Jacob replied, "Everyone on the ship addresses me as Captain. I made no exceptions for Ray."

Addressing Rachel, Jacob spoke more quietly now, a hint of entreaty in his voice. "I can't have you back on the *Sol Quest* and you know why. I can't protect you anymore."

"I'll cut and run and find another ship," Rachel insisted, her eyes flashing. "I won't be landlocked."

"You will stay here," Jacob flared, "and that's an order. You'll give this a six-month trial."

Tears streamed down Rachel's cheeks as she backed toward the door. "You're lying. You won't come back in six mon ... mon ..."

Jacob grabbed Rachel's arm and cut her off with a yell - "Stand down, sailor!"

Cynthia, alarmed, moved to stand with Simon as Rachel tried to free her arm and Jacob continued his tirade.

"I gave you an order. I'll put you in chains in the

hold of this house with half rations if I have to. I'll return in half a year if able."

For the next minute, no one spoke and no one moved.

As Simon and Cythia watched, they knew exactly what was to happen with Jacob and their niece.

The next day, Jacob sailed toward Cape Town, leaving Cynthia and Simon alone with an angry teenager.

Chapter Four
Rachel

Rachel spent the next three days camped in one of the guest rooms of the house, opening the door only to collect the food Sharron left outside her room.

When Simon came into the parlor five days after Jacob's departure, he first passed the dining room. The aroma of beef stew filled the house and he found the table set for three, just as it had been the last four nights. In the parlor, he found Cynthia sitting quietly on an upholstered armchair, sipping tea. She looked at Simon but said nothing. Blotchy eyes and a crumpled handkerchief gave away her feelings.

Simon poured himself a cup of tea, sat next to Cynthia and waited for her to talk.

"At first, you know," Cynthia said, "I thought what a wonderful and exciting challenge. Now I realize I have no idea what to do."

Simon nodded and put his hand atop Cynthia's.

"I've tried to talk to her," Cynthia whimpered, "but she won't respond. If she does, it's with a litany of coarse vulgarity. She then rolls face-down onto her pillow on the floor and stays there until I leave her room. She's unlike any girl, or even boy, I've ever encountered. I keep thinking she'll run away in the dead of night and Jacob will blame us if anything should befall her."

"I'll talk to her," Simon said.

"What could you possibly say?"

"I don't know. She's used to strict discipline. Did you see the way Jacob barked at her? I'll give it a try."

"You mustn't get violent. That would only make things worse. If I could, I would put her on a fast ship to catch up to Jacob and give her back."

Simon nodded. Both knew finding Jacob was impossible.

Simon knocked on Rachel's door and received no response. A second rap on the door received an angry, "Leave me alone."

"I'm coming in whether you like it or not," Simon said. He opened the door and entered.

Simon walked into a veritable pigsty. The bed coverings from sheets to quilt lay on the floor next to an open window with Rachel sprawled atop them. From this, Simon deduced that Rachel had been sleeping on the floor. He knocked a pile of dirty clothing off a chair and sat. "Time we had a talk."

Rachel sat up to lean against the wall under the windowsill, setting her jaw and crossing her arms. Simon sat for more than a minute, unmoving, until Rachel finally relaxed her arms and asked, "What?"

"My dear niece," Simon said calmly, "I think you expect me to say that you're on my ship now. I'm the captain and my wife is first mate and we expect you to toe the line and obey all our orders."

Rachel nodded slightly.

"That's not the way it works here," Simon said. "I'm a doctor and surgeon and I am the absolute captain when I deal with sick patients. But your aunt is the captain of this house and I better listen to her instructions when I'm home."

Rachel's face wrinkled in confusion. "I want to be on a ship. I was happy."

"We'll not hold you here," Simon said. "You may walk out the door whenever you wish and we'll not try to bring you back. But know, you'll always have a room and bed here if you want. Leave now or leave in the morning. Your choice."

"You don't mean it."

"I do. Every word."

Rachel pursed her lips thinking of the possibilities.

Simon continued, "You might even find a ship if you continue to disguise yourself successfully. But make no mistake, your sex will be discovered in time and I think you know that. Without Jacob to protect you, you will be raped by every man aboard. And when you are with child, you'll be dumped at the first port of call."

"That won't happen," Rachel hissed fiercely.

"Your father told me what already happened on the *Sol Quest,* and then about your rescue by the First Mate in Cape Town behind a pub. More importantly, he also told me you know this to be true."

Rachel shrugged as tears formed in both her eyes. "I was happy."

"So were we, before you appeared."

Rachel shrugged.

"You being here is not our fault nor yours," Simon continued, "but your father loves you, cares for your safety and saw no other way. Right now, no one in this house is satisfied. I say we, the three of us, try to find common ground and make the most of an impossible situation. Cynthia and I are willing to listen to you, if you're willing to listen to us. Maybe, just maybe, we can all be happier than we are now, which isn't very happy."

Rachel shrugged and nodded acquiescence.

"The first thing we do is eat together. Once we start talking, we might find solutions. What do you say?"

In quarter time, Rachel inched off the bed, walked past Simon, turned, and said, "I'm ready for my tot of rum."

Simon laughed. "Perhaps a sip of fine claret."

Rachel sat at the dining table and the smile on Cynthia's face brightened up the room. Simon went to the side table and retrieved a decanter of claret. He filled his glass generously and then Cynthia's.

When he approached Rachel's glass, Cynthia's smile evaporated. She stood, faced Simon and said, "Simon, don't you dare. Rachel will have no spirts of any kind in the house until she's reached her eighteenth birthday. Is that understood?"

Simon skulked back to his seat, looked at Rachel

and shrugged. “As I said, this is Cynthia’s domain.”

After Rachel devoured her portion of beef stew, Cynthia asked, “Please tell us of life on a ship. I haven’t a clue. What is your oldest memory?”

Something shifted in Rachel’s face – perhaps she was accepting her lot. In any case, she began to talk willingly, excitedly, of daring feats in high winds and sublime delicacies sampled in far-flung ports. For two hours, Simon and Cynthia sat glued to their chairs, their mouths agape in wonderment. Even Sharron stood outside the kitchen door listening to the tales.

“Your life experiences are like no other young woman’s,” Cynthia said at last. “I think I understand what you’re afraid of now. I promise I won’t let you be pigeon-holed into a life that will keep you cloistered like a nun.”

That night in their bedroom, Cynthia asked Simon, “Do you think the stories she tells are true?”

“I don’t know,” Simon said, fiddling with his sleep cap. “Each one was more fantastical than the previous. Imagine, climbing that rigging in a storm when she was only eight! As if Jacob would let her. But she tells them with such detail, it’s hard to believe they’re not true.”

“I believe our lives will be an adventure for a while, too,” Cynthia said, smiling at her husband.

The next morning, Cynthia remained home and made Rachel a proper British breakfast of two fried eggs, pork sausage, beans, toast and fried tomatoes.

“Jews don’t eat pork,” Rachel said, inspecting the plate.

“It’s important that we fit in,” Cynthia said. “Pork carried parasites in biblical times, so anything from a pig was forbidden. British pigs are safe. It’s one of the few rules we break … but tell no one. We do light the Sabbath candles and attend synagogue at least once a month. Did you keep kosher on the ship?”

Rachel laughed. “We had bacon whenever we could get it.”

After breakfast, as Cynthia sat in the parlor at a desk paying the family’s bills, she heard the front door slam. Cynthia rushed into the foyer to find Sharron.

“She walked out,” Sharron said, her face a mask of apprehension.

Cynthia gasped. “She has no suitable clothes!”

“She was wearing the same tattered togs she arrived in.”

“I guess we wait and see. She has no money that I know of and doesn’t have a clue where we are in London.”

“I’m guessing she won’t be back anytime soon,” Sharron said.

“I disagree,” Cynthia said. “Her father said she was smart. She’ll be back before supper after she’s blown off some steam. Leave the door unlocked.”

The door slammed again at 2 p.m. and Cynthia saw Rachel clump past the parlor up the stairs to her room without so much as a ‘hello.’

When Cynthia told Simon about Rachel’s slamming door exit and return, he laughed. “As long as she’s wearing the sailor’s outfit and has short hair, they’ll assume she’s a he. I don’t think she wants, needs or would accept a chaperone.”

At supper that evening, Rachel asked Cynthia, “Are you curious about where I went today?”

“No, not at all. You’re free to tell me, if you want.”

“Just getting the lay of the land,” Rachel said. “I’d need charts and a bloody compass to figure it out.”

That evening, Cynthia handed Rachel a small J. & G. Simms compass and a map of London.

The next morning, Cynthia took Rachel to her personal seamstress to start assembling Rachel a suitable wardrobe.

As the seamstress measured Rachel, Cynthia said, “You understand you cannot wear your hair cropped like a boy."

"The Cap'n told me as much," Rachel said, her mouth in a thin, rebellious line. "But I like it this way."

The seamstress came to Cynthia's rescue. "Listen to your aunt. I thought you'd been shaven as a treatment for head lice. You'll spend all your time telling people it's not true and they still won't believe you."

Within a week, Rachel had a modest amount of dresses – all of which she hated. Once home, she would immediately change into her loose-fitting linen shirts and pants from the *Sol Quest*. Then she would disappear out the door for a few hours, compass and map in. hand. Rachel never told where she had been. Cynthia, though curious, wisely asked nothing.

On Mondays and Wednesdays, Cynthia accompanied Simon to work as his surgical nurse, returning by 3 p.m. to help prepare dinner with Sharron. For the first few weeks of Rachel's stay, Simon and Cynthia wondered whether Rachel would still be there when they returned. In time, they realized that their niece had no intention of leaving.

"What are we to do with you?" Cynthia asked as Rachel tried out some of the seamstresses outfits. "You can't stay cooped up in the house every day. Would you like me to introduce you to other young people?"

"Not yet. I wouldn't know how to talk to them," Rachel said with a shrug.

"You'll learn fast enough," Cynthia said. "You might like others your own age."

"A bit longer maybe. I still have sea legs and the house rocks like a boat. I am curious about one thing."

"What's that?"

"Tell me what you do with Uncle Simon on those days you go to work," Rachel said.

"I'm a surgical nurse. Simon and I have worked together for eighteen years or so. Our whole married life.

I assist him in his surgeries."

"You actually stand there while Simon cuts people open?"

"Actually, that's exactly what I do, plus setting up the surgical instruments, handing him sutures and cutting tied knots, giving the occasional anesthetic, bandaging patients afterward, and other things as they are needed. If there's an anesthetic to be given, we'll always have another nurse or assistant."

"Might I come and observe?" Rachel asked. "I'm getting bloody bored here all day and –"

"Enough of the swearing," Cynthia interrupted. "I'd have to ask Simon, but I don't see why not."

"Sorry. A habit that's hard to break," Rachel said.

"It's got to stop. You're not on a ship anymore. Different rules." Cynthia said, crossing her arms. "We can't present you in socicty if vulgarities will pop out at any moment.

Rachel rolled her eyes. "I don't want to be presented anywhere."

"I mean it. The swearing has got to stop," Cynthia snapped with tone.

"Aye, aye, Captain. Anyway, I've seen my share of sliced arms and legs and helped the ship surgeon a time or two. Never used any anesthetics on board, but I've heard of chlorfor and ether."

"It's 'chlor-o-form' and ether. Of course. I'll ask Simon," Cynthia said, "but you can't be swearing around our patients."

"I'll try," Rachel said, with a shrug and an impish gleam in her eye. "It's just the way we talked on board. Almost every sentence had a swear word. Pass the bloody salt. That's a bitch of a gale. You're worthless as shit on a stick."

Cynthia shook her head. "Don't try. Do it."

Simon thought the idea of bringing Rachel to watch surgery brilliant. "The more things we do together will only bring us closer and closer."

The following Monday, Rachel accompanied Simon and Cynthia to the Royal London Hospital to watch two procedures from the viewing section in the amphitheater operating room. Simon removed an ovarian cyst followed by a below-the-knee-amputation. Cynthia acted as assistant in both cases.

Before the first cut, Simon looked up at Rachel from the surgical floor below. "If you are feeling faint, turn away and sit on the floor. You're free to leave if it's too much."

"I'm not going to faint. You shouldn't either," Rachel said with a smile, which brought laughter from Simon, Cynthia and the anesthetist.

During the procedure, Cynthia kept looking up at Rachel. "Are you faring alright?"

Wide-eyed, Rachel called down, "I'm amazed."

Afterward, Simon stayed to see consultations and round on post-operative patients.

On the cab ride home with Rachel, Cynthia asked, "So what did you think? Simon and I worried you might faint. More than a few invited guests, all men, have found the floor."

"At sea or in port, I've seen a few men on their arses, be it gruesome injuries or a missing finger. The ship surgeon taught me how to reduce a dislocated finger. Did that a few times. Men falling from the mainmast or going overboard and drowning, knife fights on or off the ship. Once, on the dock in Hong Kong, three men with knives, totally pissed, came at the lot of us."

Cynthia winced.

"Shall I go on?" Rachel asked.

"Without the colorful language, please. What did you think of the surgeries?"

"I loved it," Rachel said. "You and Uncle Simon work so well together. You seem to anticipate his every move before he does. He wouldn't ask for anything. He'd put out his hand and it was there. Like teamwork on the *Sol Quest* when we raise sail. Nothing needed to be said. Each of us knew not only what we had to do but what the sailor next to us had to do as well."

Cynthia laughed. "Simon has had to work with other nurses if I cannot be there. He tells me it's torture. He must do his work and mine at the same time."

"Do you think I could learn to be a surgeon?" Rachel asked.

"You could be an excellent surgeon but it's close to impossible to achieve that here, or most anywhere I know of. The medical schools in England don't believe women can be doctors or surgeons. Being a Jew makes it even more difficult. That's why Simon had to go to Strasbourg to study medicine."

"God damn it," Rachel screamed loud enough to scare the cab driver and his horse. "This makes me so angry. I couldn't be on a ship because I was born a woman. Now, I see something in medicine and surgery that intrigues me and again, I'm not allowed. There must be somewhere in this world where women have some rights."

"I've heard Italian medical schools do accept a few women," Cynthia said meekly.

Rachel said with a shrug. "I've never met my mother's family in Venice and don't wish to. I know they wanted to kill the captain because my mother wanted the freedom to make her own choices. Plus, they let it be known that they considered my parent's wedding in Morocco to be illegal and any children, meaning me, to be illegitimate."

"Simon often tells me it's a shame I couldn't have gone to medical school. Maybe in another life. You could still consider nursing. My life has been good."

"Because Uncle Simon allows you the freedom to make decisions. You told me he doesn't for other nurses."

"Yes. He's wonderful that way."

“I wonder if I became a nurse, would the Royal Navy allow me to serve?” Rachel asked.

“I don’t know but I’d doubt it. That said, I suppose anything is possible for someone like you. If not today, then perhaps tomorrow,” Cynthia said. “Let’s start with nursing and cleaning up your language.”

Rachel leaned across the carriage and kissed Cynthia on the cheek.

Surprised, Cynthia said, “What was that?”

Rachel said nothing and leaned over and kissed Cynthia again.

A moment later when Rachel wasn’t looking, Cynthia closed her eyes and touched her cheek where she’d been kissed.

That night after supper, Rachel thanked Simon for the day and kissed him on the cheek. Having been told about the kiss Cynthia received that day, Simon said only, “You’re welcome and I love you too.”

From that point onward, Rachel accompanied Cynthia to learn the art of surgical nursing.

Chapter Five
Goose

Rachel had street smarts but no formal education. Cynthia and Simon knew this would be an issue when it came to possible suitors.

"The other day, I gave her some mathematic problems," Simon said. "At least Jacob taught her those skills."

"Other than her swearing, her English is quite presentable and her penmanship impeccable," Cynthia said.

"I don't believe there are schools in England for girls her age."

"There are not. But she should have some social skills, knowledge of history and language skills such as French and German. Don't you think?"

"Most definitely."

Cynthia hired a tutor, a thirty-one-year-old spinster named Miss Leslie Brown, who would come four days a week to teach Rachel formal dancing, drawing, piano forte, singing, French and German, along with English and European history. For some odd reason, Miss Brown came with the nickname "Goose," given to her as a child when she developed whooping cough and survived.

Having a good idea of what was important, Goose dropped the piano forte, drawing and singing, feeling those to be frivolous.

Goose, a good listener, and Rachel, a story teller, adored each other from the start. Rachel absorbed her lessons, often taught as they walked in the park.

Goose knew to mix inductive and deductive reasoning with Rachel's tales on the sea, but she also allowed for the girl's feelings of abandonment by Jacob to arise. Rachel trusted Goose not to tattle on her when Rachel pushed boundaries set by Cynthia, which meant the two grew even closer.

Rachel had a vague idea of sex from listening to off-hand comments by the men on the *Sol Quest* after visiting brothels in various ports.

After being put ashore in London, Rachel asked Goose about it; the answer came back in a head shaking second.

"I know nothing of it," Goose said, "and don't ask again."

Goose became so intertwined in the family that the Romains coaxed her to move into their house as a live-in governess for the next two years. No matter how hard Goose tried, she could not rid Rachel of the occasional vulgarities.

Rachel demanded to learn to ride horseback, accompanied by Goose, who knew how to ride. Goose's lessons continued as they rode together.

After seeing the male riders, she lied to her riding instructors that her guardians had allowed her to give up riding side-saddle in favor of riding astride her horse. Rachel begged Goose to keep her secret, which she did for three months.

One day, without permission from her instructors, Rachel attempted to jump a low fence. Successful, she kept pushing her horse to clear higher and higher obstacles, until the horse declined, throwing Rachel to the ground and bruising her shoulder and forehead. Simon, seeing the bruises and getting a litany of small lies from Rachel and Goose, went directly to the stables to learn the truth. He forbade Rachel from riding for a month and demanded the instructors have her stop jumping and return to side-saddle.

Still, if Rachel went on back-country horse rides with only Goose, she would throw her leg over the side saddle and ride astride.

The effort to domesticate Rachel continued - with two steps forward and one step back.

"Your niece has both her parents' wildness in

spades," Cynthia observed to Simon, "and seems not to care a bit."

"And we both love her for it," Simon replied. "However, we must rein her in a bit or we'll never find her a husband."

Cynthia laughed and added, "Reins, indeed. I'm thinking shackles."

Chapter Six
Jacob Returns - 1852

Rachel, now eighteen, had bid goodbye to her beloved friend and teacher Goose – now off to tutor other pupils – and was working beside her aunt and uncle as a nursing student.

Under Cynthia's tutelage, Rachel learned to change bandages effortlessly and care for patients post-operatively. At night, she read books on medicine and during mealtimes she would pick Simon's brain about medical conditions she'd read about and his many surgical operations. Her curly auburn hair had grown long and radiant, she wore dresses without complaint, and she walked more and more like a lady. Sometimes she went as long as a week without mentioning how much she missed the open sea, but rarely did she go more than a day without swearing at something.

Two and a half-years after Rachel's arrival in London, Jacob, a bit more wizened, came for a week-long visit. Rachel was out shopping with Cynthia when he came to the house, so Jacob and Simon sat together for lunch.

"I can't thank you enough for the care you've provided for Ray," Jacob said, spearing an enormous bite of steak onto his fork.

"I believe Cynthia has weaned Rachel off of her sailor's name," Simon said with a smile. "She's comfortable with Rachel now. She has found a new passion in the art of surgical nursing. She has gifted hands and a soothing touch with patients. She's also quite the beauty."

"No problems?" Jacob asked, swallowing with effort and wiping his mouth.

"Her language remains colorful at times," Simon said. "But once a week now, a patient or their family asks if they can make introductions."

"How do these introductions go?" Jacob asked, his

brow darkening.

"She thinks the young men are soft and frivolous. None understand why she wastes her time becoming a nurse. All are taken aback by her colorful language at times. She tells them she has no intention of becoming serious until she's learned the art of nursing. I believe she has crushed a few hearts."

Jacob laughed heartily at this. "Then I must have taught her bloody damn well."

"Not funny," Simon replied.

"The only reason I've returned to London," Jacob said, "is to create a trust fund for Ray as my sole heir. I've no intention of marrying again and have become quite well-to-do. My money and the money from the sale of father's business has been wisely invested by the Bank of London. I will list you and Cynthia as executors. The trust will pay you fifty pounds a month to administer Ray's funds."

"Again, it's Rachel now."

"Hard for me to think of him – *her* as Rachel," Jacob lamented. "I do miss her, but I understand a life at sea would have been impossible."

"The trust fund is a wise plan," Simon consoled him, selecting a bread roll. "She'll be wealthier than me. I will tell Cynthia of the trust, but not Rachel. If suitors get wind of her wealth, they'll be queued up on our stoop in a line that extends to Manchester."

"You must tell her of the money only when you trust her to make wise decisions," Jacob said.

"Of course," Simon said. "When might you return to London?"

"It took longer for me to return to London than I told Ray and I don't plan to stay long," Jacob said. "I hope he – she – doesn't have a setback and wish to return to the sea."

Giving up on trying to get Jacob to use 'Rachel' instead of "Ray', Simon said, "I don't think so. I believe she misses you more than the sea."

That afternoon, father and daughter saw each other for the first time in more than two years.

"Is it you, Ray?" cried Jacob, embracing his daughter in a sudden flood of emotion. 'My God, is it really you?'

"It's me, Captain, it's me!" Rachel sobbed. "You said you'd be back in six months. It's four times that."

"You're the spitting image of your mother. Breathtaking to behold," said Jacob dazedly, wiping away tears. "Don't be angry with me, please. I came as soon as I could."

"I forgive you, I understand now why you left me here," Rachel said, wiping away tears. "I'm not angry with you and I've a new life now. I'm to be a surgical nurse. Aunt Cynthia has become my mentor in every way."

Jacob could only smile.

Rachel led her father to the sofa where they could converse more comfortably. "I want to know everything," she said. "How's Ol' Tom?"

"His knees have given way and he's returned to Bournemouth and family. Best first mate I've ever had, and I'll miss him. Over the years, Ol' Tom has always given me good counsel."

"I miss him too," Rachel said. "Maybe I'll visit him some day."

"He'd love that," Jacob said. "Never having had any children of his own, he considered you his child as well."

Jacob and Rachel took long walks for the next two days. They laughed and cried, recanting episodes of days past and new ones while gone from each other.

"I must leave again," Jacob said. "I miss the sea."

"As do I," Rachel said. "When will you return to London? It's been too long."

"I don't know. I've developed short, quick and well-paying routes in the Far East. I think it may be a while."

"I'll miss you," Rachel said.

"I know, as will I. I'm sorry," Jacob lamented.

Jacob never returned to London. After two years, the flow of letters stopped. A year after that, Simon and Cynthia learned from Lloyd's of London, Jacob's insurance brokers, that the *Sol Quest* had sunk in a typhoon in the Gulf of Siam.

Rachel, learning that evening of her father's demise, locked herself in her room for twenty-four hours. When she appeared at dinner the next evening, her face hollow and her eyes red, she said, "The Captain knew the risks. We all accepted them. I know he was happy doing what he did. I only hope to be so happy."

Simon held a memorial service for Jacob at his house, inviting merchants who had worked for their father and Jacob alike. Rachel, who knew Jacob far better than anyone attending, gave a lengthy eulogy for her father. Cynthia and Simon were astonished at Rachel's confidence and natural ability to orate before a group without notes.

"...Lastly, excuse me if I use sailor's terms, but that's what the Captain would expect. I called him Captain, not father. He was my best friend for almost sixteen years. You might be taken aback from the stories I've told here, assuming that the Captain wasn't a good parent. You'd be dead wrong and all at sea."

Laughter rang through the house.

Rachel continued. "I don't remember my mother, she died when I was one, so the Captain had to be both. When I turned six and joined the crew of the *Sol Quest*, I got to be with him every day for ten years. He taught me everything I needed to know to become the person I hope to become. He taught me to be strong, smart, self-sufficient, curious, and industrious. Of course, life is never all smooth sailing. The Captain used to say that a calm ocean never taught anyone to be a true sailor. The Captain taught me when to pipe down, toe the line, take the con, batten down the hatches, get out of the doldrums, run a tight ship – and when to give some a wide berth or cut and run."

Another round of laughter and smiles filled the room. Rachel had to stop to wipe the tears from her eyes. Simon rose from his seat, giving her a handkerchief and a hug. After taking a few moments to collect her thoughts, Rachel went on.

"I believe I can read the bearings on the people I meet by the cut of their jib. All things I learned from the Captain. He cut me little slack and I'm the better for it.

"But most of all, I know he loved me and did the best for me when it mattered. I hated him for forcing me to become a landlubber when he realized the ship was no place for a young woman. But he did right by having me live with my aunt and uncle. I came to realize he did it out of love. For that I will be eternally grateful. I know he died happy, doing what he loved most, being on the open sea, and knowing his daughter was in good hands, squared away and safe. Captain, I love you and always will."

At the end, not a dry eye could be found in the audience.

The night after Jacob's memorial, Simon and Cynthia told Rachel about the trust fund left by her father. Rachel seemed not to care about the fund or its importance. She promised to tell Simon and Cynthia before disclosing it to anyone else.

In the months after Jacob's memorial, Rachel occupied herself during the day by following Cynthia and Simon whenever possible and at night with reading medical and nursing texts, including a new edition of James Wilkinson's *The Human Body and its Connexion with Man.* Rachel devoured the book nightly. Just before she finished Wilkinson's treatise, Simon gave her a rare opportunity.

"My friend, Henry Gray of St. Georges Hospital, is quite the young surgeon and pathologist. He and a medical student named Henry Carter have started to create an illustrated atlas of human anatomy and they've asked me to review each printing plate for accuracy.[6] Of course I said I'd be delighted to, which gives us the opportunity to review their work together."

"Young surgeon? Medical student? Are you and Cynthia trying to find a match for me again?" Rachel asked suspiciously.

Simon laughed. "I'm afraid Gray is married and Carter's already engaged. Not to mention he isn't your type."

"What does that mean? I don't even know what my type is."

"He's a bit of a dandy," Simon said, "and quite full of himself. Unless you're thinking of only the latest fashions and hair styles, he won't take you seriously. Plus, he's a devout member of the Church of England and, daresay, not apt to court anyone whose parents are Jewish."

"No thank you, then," Rachel said.

Simon paused, speaking cautiously.

"You know every eligible medical student around has asked Cynthia or the other surgeons who is the pretty young nurse who follows me around."

"What does Aunt Cynthia say?"

"So far she hasn't liked the looks of any of them and none are Jewish," Simon said. "She says you're a guttersnipe, found on the street, and whose parents died of syphilis. That often ends the conversation."

"She doesn't say that, does she?"

"No," Simon said, "but she wishes she had

---

[6] Gray's Anatomy, now in its 42nd edition, remains even today as the quintessential textbook of anatomy.

sometimes."

"It's not so far from the truth," Rachel said, which made them both laugh.

Rachel had become the main focus of Cynthia's life. When alone, Cynthia admitted to Simon and friends that she felt very lucky, to have been given this late-arriving chance to raise a daughter. Simon voiced the same.

Cynthia and Simon spared neither expense nor time spent in Rachel's upbringing. Simon, remembering his loveless childhood in boarding school, fulfilled the pledge he had made to Cynthia's parent about being a loving and doting parent. In turn, Rachel revered her adopted parents.

Under Cynthia's tutelage, Rachel started assisting in Simon's minor surgeries and rounded with him on post-operative patients and helping in the office. Whenever Cynthia joined them, Rachel assisted with the delivery of chloroform anesthesia and became proficient quickly.

Chapter Seven
Andrew
1854

Simon left his office in the late afternoon to make a courtesy call on the elderly widow of one of his father's old trading partners. With Rachel's assistance, he had repaired the seventy-year-old woman's umbilical hernia a week earlier.

As the sun began to set, Rachel, alone in the back office, sat at Simon's desk tracing the muscles of the thigh from Gray's yet unpublished book of anatomy. Hearing a commotion in an exam room down the hall, she left the tracing and went to discover the origin of the noise.

In the hallway, staring into an examination room, stood two young men, one tall, one short, both wearing dirty cricket uniforms. They seemed to be arguing. The men stopped as Rachel approached. From within the exam room, she could hear someone muttering, "Damn it all. Damn it all ..."

Without hesitation, Rachel entered the exam room, followed by the two men. She found a handsome young man with dark, curly hair, azure eyes, and a fair complexion. He wore a cricketeer's uniform and sat on the exam table holding his left hand in the air. His ring finger was bent awkwardly backward from the middle joint up toward the back of the hand.

"Who are you and where is Mr. Romain?" the man barked. "I need a surgeon immediately."

"Mr. Romain is out making house calls," Rachel said. "He'll return in an hour or so, perhaps longer. He had no appointments this afternoon ..."

"I'm gravely injured and it hurts like hell," the curly-haired man said piteously.

"He's in frightful shape," the short cricketeer agreed. "We need him for a match in two weeks. This is awful," the tall cricketeer said.

Rachel approached the injured man, looking closely at the hand.

"Don't touch it," the man cried, withdrawing his hand to his chest.

"Stop whining! You've merely dislocated the finger. Hardly a grave injury," Rachel said. "I've seen men with their whole hand gone who don't complain half as much."

"Aren't you the cheeky one. Can I see another surgeon? I can't wait an hour."

"What's your name?" Rachel asked.

The injured man remained silent but the short man answered.

"He's Captain Andrew Drayer of the First King's Dragoon Guards. His older brother is Anthony Drayer, the Earl of Brandler." The short man pointed to tall one. "That tall lug over there is Lieutenant Kenneth Eakes and I'm Lieutenant Sam McCollum."

Sam added, "Andrew's our best bowler. We've a cricket match in two weeks against the Prince of Wales Dragoons."

"Well then, this is serious," Rachel said, shaking her head. "Here I thought the French had landed in Dover and were marching on London."

"Are you going to help me or not?" Andrew asked.

"Looks to me that you've got three options," Rachel said, arms crossed. "Go searching for another surgeon at this late hour whilst the finger swells and becomes useless. Or wait for Mr. Romain, hoping he returns soon. Or let me address it."

"How old are you? Fourteen?" Andrew asked.

"Old enough to know you've dislocated a finger and that I know how to fix it. I've seen a few," Rachel said.

"Where have you seen a few?" Andrew asked in disbelief.

"At sea, aboard a three-hundred-ton brig, but also here in Mr. Romain's office."

“You’re not a sailor. I don’t believe it,” Andrew said.

“I don’t care whether or not you believe the truth.”

“Can you actually fix this?”

“I can try,” Rachel said. “Trust me, the longer it stays dislocated the more difficult it will be to reduce and the longer the recovery will be.”

“I think I’m dreaming,” Andrew said, turning to his friends. “I walk into a surgeon’s office with my hand falling off, and I’m met by a strange, beautiful girl who acts like Admiral Lord Nelson and thinks she can fix me. I’m either damn lucky or about to make a huge mistake. What do you men think?”

“We should leave,” Sam said.

“There must be another surgeon near about,” Kenneth added.

“I disagree,” Andrew said. “She seems confident and I like that. I wish our recruits and half the junior officers had as much confidence. It can’t hurt to let her have a go at it.”

“Oh, it’ll hurt like a bitch for a moment,” Rachel cut in. “Sorry about the language. All those years at sea.”

Andrew held up his left hand. “God help me. Go ahead then and do what you need to do.”

“Captain, I think we should leave,” Kenneth said.

“I agree with Kenneth,” Sam said.

“No. I trust her. It’s remarkable, actually,” Andrew said.

“Lie down,” Rachel said as she rolled a piece of gauze. “Then you won’t faint. Bite on this so you don’t crack a tooth.” She handed Andrew the gauze roll then turned to Andrew’s friends. “Will one of you hold his other hand and one of you hold his arm above the bad finger. Tight enough so the good Captain can’t take a swing at me.”

Sam and Kenneth laughed, but Andrew did not. He laid down, and the two men positioned themselves on the right and left sides of him, holding his hand and arm. Andrew closed his eyes and grimaced as he bit down hard on the gauze roll.

"Captain," Rachel said. "Try not to fight me. I'm going to count to five. At one, I'll bend your injured finger back a little, which will hurt. Then at five I'll slide it back into joint. But only after I count to five will the pain be excruciating."

Andrew removed the roll from his mouth and said, "I swear if you weren't so pretty, I'd punch you." He then replaced and chomped down on the roll.

"You might do that anyway," Rachel said. "Here we go. One ..."

She bent the end of the dislocated joint backward a half inch.

"Ow, that hurts," Andrew mumbled through gritted teeth. His two friends grimaced as well and turned their head away, waiting for worst to come.

"Two ..."

She secured the end of Andrew's finger at the dislocation and slid it forward; it popped back into its proper place.

"We're done. Go ahead, sit up, and bend the finger," Rachel said.

Andrew sat up, spit the gauze roll into his hand, wiped tears away, shook his head, then examined his hand with dazzled eyes. He made a fist, expecting pain, then turned to Rachel. "It doesn't hurt anymore. You said it would hurt at five."

"Three, four, five. I lied," Rachel smiled.

"You're as cunning as a fox," Andrew said.

"You shouldn't use the finger until the swelling is gone," Rachel instructed. "It'll hurt less and heal quicker if you allow me to splint it. You should be able to play in two weeks if you take care."

"Anything you say, Doctor," Andrew replied.

"I'm not a doctor. Impossible for a woman to get into medical school here in England. I'm supposed to knit, sew, sing, dance, get married, and have ten children," Rachel said as she gathered a finger splint and gauze from a cabinet.

As Rachel splinted the finger with a flat wooded stick, Andrew, mouth agape, stared at her. "If I may be so bold to ask, how old are you? I hope more than fourteen."

Rachel laughed. "I'm almost twenty and I live with Mr. Romain and his wife. They're my aunt and uncle."

"May I call on you?" Andrew asked. "Or, at least, escort you to our cricket match. We'll play in your honor as you've saved the day."

"You'll need to pass muster from my aunt," Rachel said, concentrating fully on applying the splint. "To date, no one has passed. So I'd say your chances are a long shot at best."

Andrew's eyes were fixed on Rachel, their faces only eight inches away from each other.

"What exactly is a long shot?" he asked softly. "Not a term I've heard."

Rachel concentrated fully on spinning gauze around the finger and splint, binding them together. "A long shot is a naval cannon fired at great distance with little chance of finding its mark."

"Doesn't sound promising, Captain," Sam snickered.

"I'd rather bet on the horses," Kenneth added. "Then I've got a ghost of a chance."

"I'll put in a good word because you trusted me," Rachel said. "At least you're not one of the slackers my uncle has tried to introduce me to. Insufferable idiots, all of them."

Rachel finished securing the splint and looked up at a smiling Andrew. Unaware until then how close his face was to hers; she stepped back. "You're all set. Perhaps you should return next Wednesday in the afternoon to see Mr. Romain before removing the splint."

"Will you be here?" Andrew asked.

"Don't know. My aunt will be," Rachel said.

That night, Rachel told Simon and Cynthia of her meeting with Andrew and pleaded with Cynthia to allow her to see him again. Cynthia said she'd keep an open mind when she meets him.

With Simon alone later that night, Cynthia remained uncertain.

"Rachel has made no friends since her arrival," Simon said. "If the Andrew is presentable, I don't see how you can refuse her request, Jewish or not."

The following week, Simon removed Andrew's finger splint but suggested limiting the use of his hand until the cricket match. Andrew passed muster with Cynthia at the same time, and thus accepted an invitation to dine with the family.

The next evening at seven, Sharron escorted Andrew, in his dress uniform, into the study. He wore a red wool jacket with brass buttons highlighted by a striped waist-sash decked with gold and crimson tassels and embroidered boxed epaulettes denoting his rank. In one hand was a large bouquet of flowers for Cynthia and in the other, his King's Guard gilded helmet with its black plume.

Cynthia approached first.

"Ma'am," Andrew said with a bow. "A pleasure to see you again."

"Captain," Cynthia responded, "it's our pleasure and thank you for the bouquet."

Sharron took the helmet and placed it on a side table, then took the flowers and exited to find a vase. Andrew removed his gloves while Cynthia turned to Rachel. "Captain Drayer, I'd like to introduce our niece, Rachel Romain, with whom you've already had an encounter."

Simon laughed. "Knowing Rachel, it was likely hand-to-hand combat."

"Indeed," Andrew said, his eyes only on Rachel. "We were severely outnumbered, outgunned and surrounded. Only three full-grown dragoons against the impenetrable force of one young surgeon."

"I'm not a surgeon," Rachel said.

"So you said, but you had the confidence and skill of one," Andrew said. "In any event, we had no chance of victory and surrendered forthwith."

Rachel laughed and stepped forward. "The formalities are a bit much, don't you think? Come let's sit. Is your hand well?"

"Yes. Like new."

Rachel held out her hand and directed Andrew to a couch where they both sat. Simon and Cynthia took seats in upholstered chairs opposite them.

Sharron returned to announce, "Dinner will be ready in twenty minutes."

Andrew asked a question of Simon. "Rachel mentioned at our first meeting that she had been a sailor for some years. I found that hard to believe, but then this whole episode had been a fantasy. How much is real?"

"You didn't believe me?" Rachel asked.

"That's the point. I did, as your force of personality demanded it. Afterward, I didn't waver in my beliefs but my men had their doubts."

"It's all true and a bit of a saga," Simon said, "but we have a whole evening to sort it out. Rachel was raised as a boy by my brother and her seagoing name then was Ray. Only when she settled in London four years ago did she revert to her given name of Rachel."

Andrew could only shake his head and turned to Rachel. "And here I thought my life to have been interesting. I pale in your comparison."

"We all do," Simon said.

At ten p.m., Rachel walked Andrew to the door, holding his hand the entire way.

"Would you let me escort you to the cricket match on Sunday?" Andrew asked. "Our team has decided you shall be the honored guest."

"I'd be delighted, although I know little of the game,"

Rachel said.

"I'll pick you up at 1 p.m. I'll have someone sit with you to explain it all."

"Wonderful," Rachel said. She then approached Andrew, stood on her tiptoes, and kissed him on the cheek.

Stunned, Andrew said, "You just kissed me."

"I did. Am I not supposed to?" Rachel asked.

"It's certainly not the thing for a young lady called upon for the first time."

"To me, this is the second time you've called on me and that's more than enough. You trusted me when your friends did not. I'd kiss you again if I could. How else will you know that I like you already?" Rachel asked. "After four years in London, I've kissed no one else I've met here."

"I'm glad you did," Andrew said, holding her hands tightly, "although you ought not to let anyone else see you kissing strange men."

"You're not strange to me. Will you think of me until Sunday, then?"

Andrew smiled. "I'll think of nothing else."

When Rachel told Cynthia about the kiss, a thirty-minute lecture followed.

Rachel listened patiently, then said: "These are the same society rules that prevent you and me from becoming doctors. And the same that tell me how to speak, dress and act."

"Yes, I suppose they are," Cynthia said.

"Do you want my opinion?"

"No, but I believe you'll tell me anyway," Cynthia said.

"Bollocks," Rachel said, as she stood and left the room. She mumbled to herself, "Damn the rules. I'll kiss Andrew anytime I want to."

The next evening after supper, Rachel complimented Sharron for the meal and kissed her on the cheek. The kiss stunned the housekeeper. Cynthia and Simon could only shake their heads.

Before the match, each member of The First Kings Dragoon Guards cricket team introduced themselves to Rachel, thanking her for saving Andrew's finger. After the introductions, they surrounded Rachel and, in unison, yelled, "For Rachel!"

During the match, Rachel sat with Brigade Colonel Gerald Newman, the Guards' commanding officer, who explained the machinations of the game. The First Kings Dragoon Guards had not defeated the Prince of Wales Dragoons since 1848, an eight-year run of bad luck. The abbreviated-format match lasted just over three hours, with the Prince of Wales victorious once again.

Afterward, Rachel dined with the team at their barracks. Within an hour, every dragoon, save Andrew, was roaring drunk. Andrew, wanting to avoid an embarrassing incident, escorted Rachel home early.

"I'm sorry for my friends. Drowning in their misery," Andrew said.

"You think I haven't seen men groggy? I used to think that was their normal state," Rachel said.

"I bet you have," Andrew replied with a smile.

"Do you want to know the reason why I'm no longer aboard a ship?" Rachel asked.

"No. I can only guess."

"It's because my father couldn't guarantee my safety when the men had too much rum," Rachel said. "Thank you for leaving and staying sober. I had a marvelous time."

"I know cricket isn't your fancy," Andrew said, "and I'll be occupied with training recruits for the next week. After that I have some free time. Can you ride?"

"I believe I'm quite good at it."

"Would you like to go riding with me?"

"I'd love it."

"Do you need to get permission from your aunt?"

Andrew asked as they stood at Rachel's front door.

"No. I'll tell her. Also, I care little for society norms and fashions. I refuse to ride side-saddle like other women. If I could wear my sailing trousers, I would. I won't because I don't want to embarrass you."

Andrew laughed and said, "Wear what you want. It's all fine by me. I'll pick you up Friday after next at 9 a.m. but I'll need to be back at the barracks for dinner."

This time, Rachel stood on tiptoes and kissed Andrew softly on the lips.

Andrew escorted Rachel, in a dress, to ride in Hyde Park and brought a picnic lunch. They talked of Rachel's time at sea and Andrew's need to join the army to make a living.

That night at dinner with her aunt and uncle, Simon asked, "So, how was it?"

"I had a wonderful time," Rachel said. "Andrew is quite the gentleman and as you'd expect from a dragoon, an excellent horseman. I enjoy his company. Next Wednesday, we'll ride in Richmond Park and then go to dinner. Then Sunday we'll ride in Trent Park."

"I'm happy for you," Cynthia said.

"He's my first real friend here, man or woman," Rachel reflected. "He applauds my wish to be a nurse. I would spend every day with him if I could."

"There are other men," Simon said. "You need to broaden your scope. Does he know you're Jewish?"

"Of course," Rachel said. "It bothers him not at all. Nor does it bother me that he's not."

"Not yet, anyway," Cynthia said.

Rachel shrugged at the comment.

After their last ride at Trent Park, Andrew escorted Rachel home. At the door, he said, "I'm planning an outing for us in two weeks that I believe you'll love."

"Tell me more?"

"Let me get things sorted first," Andrew said. "I don't want to get your hopes up. It involves leaving London for a long weekend."

"I'd have to clear that kind of outing with Aunt Cynthia. I may require a chaperone," Rachel said. "A deal we struck as long as I live in their house."

"I'm happy to have you chaperoned if that's what it takes," Andrew said. "If it's a go, you'll not want to miss this."

"Please tell me," Rachel begged. "Patience is not one of my strong points."

"Don't I know."

"Then tell me."

"No. Not 'til it's set. Once it's done, I'll break free and explain the particulars to you and your aunt and uncle."

At the door of her house, Rachel turned to Andrew. "I had the most marvelous time. I can't wait to hear about our possible outing."

"And I can't wait to see you again. You're like no one I've ever met," Andrew said, taking both of Rachel's hands and bringing her close.

"I am the odd duck. Even my aunt thinks so," Rachel said, then stood on tiptoes to kiss Andrew on the lips.

Andrew swung his arms around Rachel's waist to bring her closer and the kiss lasted until Rachel needed to catch her breath.

Rachel, back on the ground, inhaled deeply, smiled and said, "That tells it all." She turned and entered her house.

Once the door shut, she smiled and mumbled, "I believe I will marry this man."

At 9 p.m., a week later, the Romains were finishing a late supper when a loud rapping on the door interrupted the meal. A minute later, Sharron escorted Andrew into the dining room wearing dirt-stained, battle clothing.

Rachel, hearing Andrew's voice, was already standing. "I see you've dressed for dinner."

Andrew laughed. "I was in the saddle with recruits but moments ago. I rode over and have only a minute to explain next weekend. I can't stay."

"We must know," Cynthia said, "what plans you have for Rachel. I won't let her go anywhere willy-nilly without some guarantees."

"Of course," Andrew said. "I'd expect nothing less. But when she hears of my plans, I doubt anyone could stop her."

"Go on then," Simon said.

"My sister-in-law, Olivia Lipson-Drayer, the Countess Brandler, has given us a rare opportunity. Her family, the Lipsons from Southampton, have generations in boat building and service in the Royal Navy. Knowing how Rachel misses the open sea, I asked the Countess if she had any suggestions. I was merely hoping for an afternoon sailing on one of their yachts. She said she'd get back to me."

"That was sweet of you," Cynthia said.

"I'd love that," Rachel said.

"However, two days ago she made me an unbelievable proposition," Andrew said. "Not at all what I expected."

"So, what is it?" Simon demanded impatiently. "Rachel cannot go back to sea for a prolonged voyage."

Andrew smiled at Rachel. "Come hold my hand whilst I explain."

Rachel obliged.

"The countess has offered me a sloop to race on the Solent around the Isle of Wight in the yearly Cowes Week Regatta. Her family had already registered the boat and paid the entrance fees but their hired skipper and his seven-man crew have defected to another boat. She knows full well we have no chance of winning, as few of my company know much about boat racing. She doesn't know we have Rachel, who will need to revert to Ray, to lead us. Women are not allowed in the races. At best we place, at worst, we'll have some fun."

"At worst, you'll all drown," Simon said, frowning. "I think it foolish. I won't allow it."

"Foolhardy," Cynthia added, exchanging a rapid glance with Simon. "We've all heard of sunken boats and men lost on the Solent."

"If the weather is foul, we'll return to shore or not leave port," Andrew said. "I won't risk anyone's life."

Rachel spun around to face her uncle. "When I first arrived, you told me I was free to leave at any time. I must do this. Andrew will see me home safe."

"Plus, we'll have a skilled and trained nurse on board for any mishaps," Andrew said.

"This is lunacy," Simon said.

For a long moment, no one spoke.

"I don't wish to start a family feud. I'm sorry if I have," Andrew said contritely. "I was hoping all of you would be excited."

"How many in the crew?" Rachel asked.

"Eight men in total are allowed. I've found five of my officers who have been on sloops, including my good friends, Lieutenants Eakes and McCollum. That's six. Seven with Rachel. We'll have room for one more."

"One more! How far is Bournemouth from Southampton?" Rachel asked.

"Thirty miles or so," Simon said. "A hundred miles from London. What does that have to do with this craziness?"

"If we're lucky, I've the eighth man," Rachel said with a huge smile. "And he can serve as my chaperone."

"Who?" Andrew and Cynthia demanded in unison.

"My father's trusted first mate, Ol' Tom Voz," Rachel said. "He retired the last time father was here but, if still able, he could captain a pig trough through a hurricane. If not him, he'll know someone."

"How will you find him?" Simon asked.

"Anyone in Bournemouth will know the Voz clan," Rachel said. "He was a cabin boy for Nelson at Trafalgar. Ol' Tom's stories are legends. I'll leave this week and meet you in Southampton."

"If you can wait until Wednesday, I'll go with you,"

Andrew said. "I'll arrange separate rooms at a hotel. The race will be on Sunday."

"Perhaps Goose, if available, can chaperone you," Cynthia said.

"Not likely," Simon added, "as I've heard she's moved to Birmingham."

"I'll be fine with Ol' Tom, Andrew and his men to escort me," Rachel said. "End of discussion."

After a lull of silence, Rachel added, "Do we still have my sailing clothes from when I arrived?"

"Sadly, I do," Cynthia said. "Please don't tell me you're going to cut your hair down to the nub."

"Only short enough to hide under a sailor's cap."

Chapter Eight
Solent #1

The following Wednesday morning, Rachel and Andrew boarded a train on the western outskirts of London for Salisbury, then caught a side line to Bournemouth, arriving at dusk. Rachel, smartly dressed, hair down, traveled as a married woman, borrowing a wedding band from Cynthia. Travel was much easier as Mr. and Mrs. Drayer – a thought that Rachel enjoyed.

In Bournemouth, the dense smell of saltwater and the annoying squawking of sea gulls hovering around fishing boats put a smile on Rachel's face.

"The sounds are music to my ears," Rachel said as she took Andrew's hand.

They hailed a cab to the Royal Bath Hotel, a seaside resort. At the hotel desk, Andrew booked two rooms, which gave the desk clerk some pause. Rachel asked for directions to pubs near the docks.

That evening, after a quick dinner in the hotel's restaurant, Andrew and Rachel, dressed casually, took a cab to a pub called the Dancing Jug near the Bournemouth docks, hoping to start the search for Ol' Tom. The shabby pub was filled with aged sailors, drunkards, rapscallions, and riff-raff. All bloodshot eyes turned to the unlikely couple as they entered.

Rachel approached the bartender with Andrew trailing.

"Oi, not my usuals. You be lost?" the bartender asked.

"Not at all," Rachel said. "A tot of rum for me and a pint of ale for my friend. Don't even think of adding lime juice to my rum.[7] I want it straight."

"Aye, Aye, Cap'n," the bartender laughed at a most unusual order from a young woman. He returned in a

---

[7] In 1795, the Royal Navy required the addition of lemon or lime juice to prevent scurvy.

minute with a pint of ale, an empty glass and a bottle of Foursquare Rum. The bartender poured exactly two and a half ounces into the empty glass.

"Might I direct a question to your fine patrons?" Rachel inquired after her first sip.

"The floor is yours, m'lady," the bartender said.

Rachel turned and found all the men watching her except those too drunk to lift their heads off the tables.

"Do any of you know Ol' Tom Voz? Raise your hand if so."

Every hand in the pub went up, including the bartender's.

Andrew laughed as Rachel turned to him and said, "What did I tell you."

Ten minutes later, Rachel had a rough address and directions. They finished their drinks and headed back to their separate rooms at the Royal Bath Hotel.

The next morning, Rachel and Andrew headed to Seward Avenue, entered the service street behind a fine home, and knocked on a ramshackle abode which sat between two stables. The smell of sewage, urine, and rotting horse manure could not be avoided.

A large, muscular man of about twenty-five answered the knock and stood speechless at the sight of an apparent gentleman and lady. Rachel smiled. The man was the spitting image of Ol' Tom, only larger and younger. She didn't wait for the young man to come to his senses before speaking.

"Excuse me, but is Ol' Tom Voz here?"

"Yeah, but he don't owe no money to no one," the man said, his eyes shifting uneasily from Rachel to Andrew.

"It's not about money. I need to speak to him," Rachel demanded.

The man turned about and yelled, "Pa, there's a lady with a gentleman says she needs to speak to you."

From another room came an answer. "I dunna know any bloody ladies or gentlemen in these here parts. Tell 'em to shove off."

Rachel knew Ol' Tom's voice like she knew her own. She yelled over the shoulder of the stunned man at the door as she walked around him into the house. "Ol' Tom, get off your fat arse and come to the door, you lazy son-of-a-bitch. You can't leave me high and dry. You owe me two tots of rum and I mean to collect."

Ol' Tom appeared seconds later, limping as fast as he could. Tom had aged a bit in two years, with sparse gray hair, wrinkled face and a bit of a stoop. Within seconds, Rachel saw none of that.

Following him was a large, buxom woman with poorly dyed red hair, wearing nothing but a tattered camisole which left little to the imagination.

Ol' Tom shouted as he approached, "Well shiver me timbers. I know that nagging Ray voice. I wondered if you'd ever shake a leg and come to see me."

Rachel rushed past the man at the door and the two old friends embraced.

"Oi, Ray, it's good to see you," Ol' Tom cried. "I'm so sorry 'bout the Cap'n and the *Sol Quest*. I ne'er would've let that happen. But what's happened, happened. I'm glad you weren't there. Oi, it's good to see you."

"You have no idea how I miss you and the open sea," Rachel said, her eyes wet with emotion.

"Ol' Tom stood back a step. "Lemme look at ya. You be an image of your ma, I swear. A grown woman and as pretty as a sunset in a calm sea."

Ol' Tom turned to the young man who had greeted Rachel at the door. "This be my son Little Tom. Didn't know he existed 'til I left the *Sol Quest*. This be his ma, Betty. Betty be a good cook among her other boons."

Ol' Tom pinched Betty's rear end, receiving a hand slap.

"Little Tom's a good lad and takes proper care of me. He's not too little, eh," Ol' Tom went on. "The Cap'n did right by me and the Bank of London sends me a pension every month. Nuf' to keep the three of us above water."

Rachel turned to Betty. "Mrs. Voz, a pleasure to meet you."

Betty let out a huge belly laugh. "I ain't never married this toad of a man. Had his kid. That's enough. Name's Betty Baugh but if you want to call me Mrs. Voz, that be fine with me."

Ol' Tom spoke up, "Betty, Tom, this here be Ray Romain, the best cabin boy and shipmate e'er, 'cept she's not a boy. Now I gotta figure why she's come a calling."

Rachel said, "I came because I need you at the helm of a ship for one more day."

"I'm too old for that. My knees are shot. Big ships are for young men," Ol' Tom said.

"I'm talking the bloody Cowes Week Regatta this weekend in Southampton," Rachel said.

"Ya don't say," Ol' Tom exclaimed, stroking his chin. "Is the Queen offering a hundred guineas agin' for the cup?"

"Yes. But don't say no until you've heard what we're about," Rachel said. She turned to Andrew. "This is Captain Andrew Drayer of the First King's Dragoon Guards. He doesn't know a mizzenmast from a bloody jib, but he and I need a captain for a day. Might we take you, Betty and Little Tom out for a pint and a bite to eat to explain it all?"

"I'll ne'er turn down food and ale," Ol' Tom said. "I see you've let your hair grow. I knew you'd be a pretty one. Still have a foul mouth. I thought for sure the Cap'n's kin would beat it outta you."

"I only talk that way with old salts like you," Rachel said. "Then they know I mean business."

The next afternoon, Rachel, Andrew, and Ol' Tom' took the train to Southampton. Andrew escorted Rachel and Ol' Tom to the Canute Castle Hotel, which was only a short walk from the docks.

Andrew sat with Rachel and Ol' Tom in the hotel lobby for a few minutes. "I have to dine with my sister-in-law, the countess, tonight. It's her boat and she's paid the fees. I'll not tell her you'll dress as a boy for the races or that you're even here in Southampton. I believe we'd never leave the dock if she or the yacht club knew the truth of it. You'll get to meet the countess at the ball Sunday evening."

"Not quite fair, is it, me being a girl and having to hide it?" Rachel asked.

Andrew nodded but didn't answer, knowing how Rachel felt.

Andrew then went to the Southampton Naval base, where he found the five officers from his company of the First King's Dragoon Guards billeted in barracks, courtesy of the Royal Navy. Once settled, he dressed formally then went to dine at the Southampton home of Lord Gerald Lipson, the brother of his sister-in-law, Olivia Lipson-Drayer, the Countess Brandler.

The Fifth Earl of Brandler, Jonathan Drayer, inherited a title, lands and money in 1805. Over the next three decades he philandered his fortune.

When he died, he left his title but insurmountable debt to his oldest son, Anthony, the Sixth Earl of Brandler. The other two brothers, Philip and young Andrew, only fifteen, received nary a farthing.

Philip had become a missionary in India, knowing that he would receive no money.

Anthony married well to Olivia Lipson and the Lipsons infused enough capital into the marriage to save the earldom. With the Lipson's capital and shrewd management, Anthony and Olivia restored the earldom. Andrew lived with his older brother, the earl and Olivia. Anthony paid for Andrew's schooling then his commission into the Royal Army.

Olivia, now forty yet still striking, tall, with black hair and large brown eyes, exuded intelligence, power and class. She adored Andrew and felt sorry he'd never amount to much unless he excelled in the army. Two healthy sons and a daughter already born to Anthony and Olivia settled the earldom's future without Andrew in it.

As they dined alone, Olivia pried Andrew for information. "Your brother tells me you've met a girl under the most curious of circumstances. Tell me of her."

Andrew swallowed and patted his mouth discreetly with a napkin.

"I dislocated my finger playing cricket," he said, his eyes sparkling. He was very fond of Olivia too, and enjoyed sharing confidences with her. "My sergeant knew of a surgeon nearby near Spitalfields, a Mr. Simon Romain, and off I went."

"I don't know him and I thought I knew every surgeon of import in London," Olivia said, her brow furrowed.

"He has a nice and well-appointed office but was out making house calls," Andrew said. "His niece, Rachel, works as his nurse and assistant. It was she that put my finger right, almost painlessly. She splinted the finger and when I saw Mr. Romain a week later, the finger was as good as new."

Andrew put down his fork and wiggled his fingers to prove the point.

"This is the woman you're courting?" Olivia asked. "A nurse for her uncle?"

"Yes. She's quite remarkable. Like no one I've ever encountered."

"Near Spitalfields, you say, and her name is Rachel. She's a Jew, my dear Andrew. That's why I know little of Mr. Romain," Olivia said with a subtle shrug.

"I know. What of it?" Andrew asked. "You'll like her. Mr. Romain and his wife were most gracious when I dined with them. Religion wasn't brought up. They hadn't the trappings of the religious Jews with the black caps and long sideburns."

"Ridiculous," Olivia said, her cheeks flushing. "A Jewess with a job? So beneath you, the son of an earl! You know how fond I am of you, how much I encourage you to forge your own path, but this is truly out of the question. I'd suggest ending your dalliance if you expect to get anywhere in the Royal Army. Besides, if you don't end it, the army will."

Andrew stiffened. He has never found himself at odds with Olivia before.

"She arrives Sunday morning and will attend the ball on Sunday evening as my guest," he said woodenly. "I hope you will extend every courtesy to her for the weekend."

"To what end?" Olivia demanded. "Why lead the poor girl on?"

Andrew reached for his wine and took a long, fortifying sip.

"Please meet her before you feed her to the wolves. Besides, I've heard rumors our regiment will be sent to the Far East to help quash an uprising among the Punjabi locals. I've not told Rachel and won't until it's definite. If I go abroad, I believe our relationship will end."

Olivia sat back, still simmering but somewhat satisfied, and reached for her own wine glass.

"It had better," she said. "Let's speak of more pleasant matters. Tomorrow, before the race starts, I'd like to greet the crew of our yacht, the *Glory B,* which will be sailing under the Lipson banner."

"Of course," Andrew said, "and thank you again for allowing us to participate. Tomorrow, our crew will learn the boat."

"I trust you have sourced at least one competent man who knows how to handle a sloop?"

"We've one very experienced sailor," Andrew said, "who will captain us. He's brought his young nephew along who knows the ropes."

"I sincerely hope that all of you can swim."

"All of us are comfortable in the water."

"Good. You may need it. I'll never understand why a group from the Royal Army with little to no sailing experience wants to take on this race. But if it makes you happy, then I am delighted."

Andrew departed his aunt's company that night with an uneasy feeling in his stomach. He didn't want his relationship with Rachel to end – but he saw now that many forces could converge to make it so.

The next morning, Ol' Tom and Rachel, dressed as a boy, snuck out a side service door of the Canute Castle Hotel. Walking a few blocks, they waited outside the Royal Yacht Squadron gates. The mid-August day was warm and sunny with a ten to twelve knot south-westerly wind. They wore the same clothing they had worn as crew on the *Sol Quest* - baggy trousers and linen shirts with drawstrings at the neck. Rachel had purchased a wide gauze roll and Ol' Tom tightly wrapped her chest over a camisole to conceal her breasts as best he could. She had coiled her hair in a tight bun and wore an oversized flat cap to conceal it.

Minutes later, Andrew and his five dragoons arrived, wearing matching cotton shirts and trousers with leather boots. They all knew Rachel from the cricket match and that she would be dressed as a boy.

Andrew laughed at Rachel's disguise. "Indeed, you look like a twelve-year-old boy. Where has your chest gone?"

Rachel said with a smile, "I left it in the hotel room."

Andrew's friends, Kenneth Eakes and Sam McCollum could barely stop from laughing at Rachel's transformation.

"Enough of that from you four. We got work to do," Ol' Tom interrupted, "and gotta see what we're sailing." He then addressed the dragoons. "First thing, all you landlubbers need to get those bloody boots off. Sailors work in bare feet. The first minute on a wet deck and you'll know why."

The eight-man crew, boots in hand, approached the *Glory B,* a single-masted, narrow-beamed, deep-drafted, forty-four-foot sloop. She was rigged fore-and-aft, which meant the sails were set along the line of the keel and not perpendicular like the typical square-rigged ship. She sported a triangular mainsail set from the mast toward the aft, which could be spread with a boom and jibs set from the forestays. The *Glory B* exuded speed.

Standing in front of the ship, Ol' Tom addressed Rachel, Andrew and the five dragoons. "My name is Ol' Tom and I am your Cap'n. I run a tight ship. Tighter than a duck's arse. My first mate here is Ray. He's an able seaman and you may know him by another name. Forget what you knew. It's Ray. When I give a command, you respond, 'aye, aye, Cap'n, that you've heard it, then do it. Got it?"

Ol' Tom waited for the dragoons to respond, which they did in one, loud voice: "Aye, aye, Captain."

"Good," Ol' Tom continued. "Today, I will try to teach you the ropes. We didn't come here to look pretty and lose this race. Understood?"

"Aye, aye, Captain," the dragoons yelled.

Rachel grabbed Ol' Tom's hand as he led the dragoons on board. "Oh, how I've missed the sound of your voice giving orders," she said. "I feel like I'm back on the *Sol Quest* cruising the South China Sea."

Ol' Tom nodded, then smiled. "I'd forgotten how much I missed it as well."

With the dragoons following, Ol' Tom began by naming and explaining the parts of the *Glory B,* starting with basic terminology and purposes: Fore, aft, port, starboard, mainsail, jib, deck, lines, boom, rigging, shrouds, ratlines, and rudder.

As Ol' Tom lectured, Rachel wandered away. She took in the pungent odor of old wood, pine tar, hemp, linseed oil, tallow, and turpentine as she ran her hands along the shrouds and railings. She whispered to herself, "I'm home." Comforted, she returned to hear the rest of Ol' Tom's instructions.

Ol' Tom laid down ground rules for the crew once again. "I am the Cap'n and what I says goes. If I tell any of yous to do something, you don't argue or discuss it – you say 'aye, aye, Cap'n,' and do it. Understood?"

"Aye, aye. Captain."

"If Ray tells you to do something, you do it. Ray's forgotten more than you'll ever know. If Ray says, 'pull,' you pull. If Ray says, 'loosen a line', you loosen it. If Ray says 'move,' you move. If Ray says 'piss,' you piss. No questions. Understood?"

"Aye, aye. Captain."

"Off the boat, Cap'n Drayer resumes command. Ray, do you have anything to add?"

"No, Cap'n."

"Good. I went to a pub last night," Ol' Tom continued, "and heard scuttlebutt from Royal Navy men about a raggedy-ass group of Royal Army dragoons scraped from the bottom of a shithole who plan to race in the Cowes Week Regatta. They were betting how many of you would drown or scream for your mothers. Winning was out of the question. I'm here to prove 'em wrong."

The looks on the faces of the men showed Ol' Tom that he had struck a chord. These men were eager to put up a fight.

Andrew also sensed it. He pulled a pennant with the colors of the King's Dragoons from a satchel and raised it over his head. The men cheered in unison.

"Captain," Andrew asked, "may we put our King's Guard pennant under the Lipson pennant?"

"I'm all fer it," Ol' Tom said. "Give it to Ray."

Without hesitation, Rachel grabbed the pennant, stuck it in under her rope belt, effortlessly climbed the ratlines to the top of the mainsail, and attached the pennant. She came down at double speed. To a man, the

Dragoons were cured of any suspicion that Rachel hadn't been a sailor. Ol' Tom hardly noticed.

"I guess you *were* raised on a ship," Andrew said faintly. "I've no words." He turned to his friends, Eakes and McCollum, and added, "You two were dead wrong."

Both nodded in defeat.

Ol' Tom wasted no time getting the *Glory B* out to sea through the Southampton Water inlet, setting sail around the Solent, the strait between the mainland and the Isle of Wight. Ol' Tom and Rachel spent the day barking orders at the men. They could barely speak by the time they headed back to their hotel.

Ol' Tom rasped, "What'ja think?"

"Better than expected," Rachel whispered back. "They want to win."

"A long shot," Ol' Tom said. "A very long shot. But I love the odds."

"Put me in for five pounds," Rachel said. "It's good to sail with you again."

"And you, Ray," Ol 'Tom averred, his voice cracking. "The Cap'n would be proud to see you now."

The next morning at 9 a.m., the crew of the *Glory B* met Olivia at the dock. She shook the hands of each sailor, including Rachel, who kept her face down and her voice lowered, saying only, "Ma'am."

"Your name, young man?" Olivia asked.

"Ray Voz, Ma'am."

Olivia then addressed the men. "Good luck to you all and may the wind always be at your backs. I pray you will return safely, but I would be most pleased if you could beat the yacht from the Liverpool Yacht Club who stole my crew only a month ago."

"For Olivia," Andrew yelled, facing his men.

"For Olivia," the crew yelled back.

With that, the Dragoons, Rachel and Ol' Tom boarded the *Glory B* and took her into the Solent to await the 10 a.m. cannon shot that would start the race around the Isle of Wight in a counterclockwise direction. Eight additional sloops had entered the race, including one owned by Queen Victoria and Prince Albert, and others from the Royal Yacht clubs of Liverpool, Southampton, Edinburgh, Dublin and three from London.

At the cannon shot, the race began.

Having spent hours in the pubs talking to old crews and weathered seamen, Ol' Tom had a few tricks up his sleeve. Lacking mobility, Ol' Tom stayed at the helm and barked commands to Rachel. She then would scurry about the sloop, relaying and implementing the commands.

Once into the Solent, Tom headed the *Glory B* west-southwest toward the Sconce Point buoy to use the tides rushing into the English Channel. From there, he set a course due east for Hurst Castle off the mainland. With the winds against him to the southwest, Ol' Tom found a current near the Shingles off the Needles Isle and passed two sloops out in deeper water. Coming around the east end of the Isle of Wight, the *Glory B* held second place, only a half a boat behind the sloop from the Royal Dublin Yacht club.

Ol' Tom tacked hard to the starboard to establish a position windward of the Irish boat, putting them in the *Glory B's* wind shadow. The Irish sails became slack with no wind to fill them, and ended up dead in the water. Not until the *Glory B* was well past them would their sails fill, but by then it would be too late to make up lost ground. All the men aboard the *Glory B* cheered, in high spirits.

By this time, the tides were rushing into the Solent. Ol' Tom engineered a fast, high approach on a starboard tack and won the race by twelve minutes.

A thousand spectators with spyglasses and binoculars watched the Dragoons screaming and hugging in delight on the *Glory B's* deck. Rachel scampered up and down the ratlines to retrieve the

King's Guard Dragoon pennant, which each man raised over their heads with a cheer. In a fit of joy, Andrew lifted Rachel, kissed her, then spun her around, causing her cap to fly off, releasing her hair down to her mid-back. The men surrounded Rachel as she restuffed her cap.

"I shouldn't have spun you about and I fear you've been spotted. As soon as we dock, you'll need to make yourself scarce," Andrew said, his face ashen, fearing discovery and disqualification.

"I'll take her back to the hotel," Ol' Tom cut in. "If anyone asks, tell 'em his ma needed us home and we caught the evening train."

The moment the Glory B docked, Rachel and Ol' Tom disembarked. Rachel raced off the pier, running by the exuberant countess without saying a word. Olivia raised a hand to stop her, but on she ran. Trying to keep up with Rachel, Ol' Tom limped past Olivia moments later without stopping.

Olivia seemed annoyed, but she only shrugged her shoulders and continued toward the *Glory B*. She was far too happy to complain, as her ship had won the cup. Better yet, the Liverpool yacht and its faithless crew could not be seen on the horizon. They would finish an hour later.

Once clear of the docks and spectators, Rachel stopped and waited for Ol' Tom. Both wore smiles from ear to ear, as Rachel jumped into his arms.

"Oi, Ray," Ol' Tom cried, "I wished the Cap'n' was here. He'd be so proud. I'm gettin' too old to keep you in the air like I used to." He put Rachel back to the ground.

Rachel sniffled. "What makes you think he's not watching from above. I can feel it."

"Spose, you be right. You best get goin' back to the hotel and change your look. I'd go through the side door agin."

"Where'll you be," Rachel asked, knowing full well Ol'

Tom’s first stops.

“Gotta see some old sea dogs ‘bout some money they owe us. You have a good time tonight. My uncle married a Scots lassie. She used to say Whit's fur ye, nae go by ye.”

Rachel squiggled her nose, “What’s that supposed to mean.”

Ol’ Tom smiled, “I think it’s meant to say, ‘Don't let what's for you go by you.’”

Rachel shrugged, still not sure about the saying’s meaning. Both laughed and went on their way.

Chapter Nine
Olivia

That night at the Regatta Ball, the Dragoon officers came in full dress uniforms, while Rachel was resplendent in an emerald-green evening gown that revealed her neck and shoulders, with a single lace rose at the neckline. The skirt was pattered with rose bouquets and replete with flounces and ten petticoats.

Olivia had arranged female escorts from Southampton's finest families for Andrew's men.

As Rachel and Andrew entered the ballroom, she said, "You know you're quite handsome in your dress uniform."

"There's not a man here not jealous of me now," Andrew said.

"Because you won the cup?" Rachel asked.

"No. Because I'm with you. You will be the prettiest woman in the hall."

"Would they think that if they knew how I detest wearing this dress."

Andrew laughed, then said, "First, I must introduce you to the countess. A huge hurdle. You must act as yourself."

Andrew had not told Rachel of the tense conversation with Olivia the evening before and seemed out of sorts.

Rachel sensed Andrew's anxiety from the beads of sweat on his forehead. "Are you okay? Are you worried about me meeting the countess? You needn't be. I can handle myself." Rachel lied, she was scared stiff.

"You are something else," Andrew responded with a smile, trying to hide the knot in his chest.

Arm in arm, Andrew walked Rachel off to find the countess.

Olivia excused Andrew as soon as he introduced Rachel.

"You will excuse us, won't you, Andrew darling," Olivia said. "Go find your men and celebrate. I must talk to Rachel alone."

Andrew had no option other than to retreat, head down, leaving the two alone.

Rachel, her lip quivering, only shrugged and faced Olivia. "Congratulations on your victory. You must be pleased with Andrew."

"Yes. Yes, I am," Olivia said. "You're certainly a pretty one. My young brother-in-law seems quite smitten with you. He's told me of your nursing prowess."

"I'm quite fond of Andrew as well," Rachel replied with a smile, relaxing at the light conversation. "Quite an odd way to meet. Him moaning in pain with an immobile finger and me chiding him about it. He then met with my aunt to arrange a formal introduction."

Olivia stared at Rachel's face as they talked, then held her thumb and index finger in a circle to outline her face. Her actions confused Rachel but Olivia smiled at the result. "Did you arrive today from London?"

"Yes. On the afternoon train," Rachel lied.

"I can't help but notice your windblown complexion. Did you spend the entire train ride with your face out the window?" Olivia asked.

Stunned, Rachel stammered, "Oh. Um, of course not." Her ploy had not fooled Olivia.

Olivia folded her arms. "My dear, you understand that if you tell the truth, you never have to remember what you've said. Andrew tells me you are indeed unique. I'd say he's got that right." She looked at Rachel expectantly, waiting for a confession.

"You won't tell, will you?"

"That it was you and the *Glory B* skipper that galloped by me on the dock after the race?"

Rachel acknowledged her guilt with the tiniest nod.

"I thought so. Actually, quite smart of you. You understand you shouldn't have been on the ship and we could have been disqualified?"

Rachel nodded again. "You won't tell?"

"Of course not, Ray Voz or Rachel, whoever it is," Olivia said. "Winning the race means a great deal to my family. I won't take that away. Quite remarkable and impressive."

"Thank you," Rachel said.

"You're welcome, but you must know that I have told Andrew to discard you."

Said in a flat, emotionless, matter-of-fact tone, the comment stunned Rachel as if Olivia had punched her hard in the stomach. She held her hand to her mouth for a moment and swallowed hard. "Why, may I ask?"

"You're a Jewess, of course."

It was a statement, not a question. Rachel answered anyway. "Yes. What of it?"

"Andrew will never amount to anything in the Royal Army with a Jewess for a wife. Worse, he hasn't the funds to be anything outside the army. That's why the Earl and I will advise Andrew to discard you. I expect Andrew to follow our advice." Olivia waited, expecting Rachel to crumble. She misjudged Rachel.

Rachel tightened her jaw and held her head high, refusing to show weakness. "Say what you will, Andrew won't relinquish me, nor will I him. I've got the wind at my back."

Rachel's strong response surprised Olivia who blinked hard. "I may be wrong about you," she mused. "I saw you climb the ratlines on the *Glory B* to retrieve the Dragoon pennant like a sailor born and bred on a ship."

Rachel kept her face impassive.

"How does a pretty Jewish nurse from London know her way around a sloop? Quite remarkable." Olivia continued softly. "You certainly are a mystery, and mysteries don't sit well with me. I like to be in the know. Yes, I'd like to know more of you before I force Andrew's hand. I believe you and I should have a luncheon in London."

"As you wish," Rachel said.

"I'll have my secretary arrange something. Yes, I'd like to know more of you. Now go off and enjoy your victory with my brother-in-law."

For the rest of the evening, congratulations flowed from every corner of the ballroom, including a bow and curtsy in front of Queen Victoria and Prince Albert. Everyone wanted to know who skippered the *Glory B*, and whether a young woman had been on board the yacht. Andrew and the dragoons refused to divulge the captain's name and insisted the deckhand was Ray, the nephew of the mysterious captain.

Meanwhile, Olivia was so excited over the victory that she gave the one-hundred guinea prize to Andrew to be distributed amongst the crew. Rachel smiled and did her best to act happy, although her conversation with the countess had left a feeling in her stomach akin to spreading poison.

After the Queen and Prince Albert left the floor, the band played the first waltz. Andrew and Rachel were invited, with great applause, to dance alongside the Commodore of the Royal Yacht Squadron and his wife. Soon the rest of the guests joined them.

As they danced, Rachel revealed the details of her conversation with Olivia. "The countess figured out I was Ray."

Andrew tripped slightly but recovered quickly.

"How?" he demanded.

"She noticed the color on my face from being in the sun and wind all day and knew I'd been at sea. Have you forgotten already that you kissed me in front of the entire crowd and my cap came off? It's a miracle more people haven't figured it out."

Andrew shook his head as if to clear it. "This whole day has been a blur."

Rachel took a deep breath. "Olivia also told me that she has advised you to discard me if you want to advance in the Royal Army."

Andrew's face grew solemn. "Yes," he said. "She is

worried about you being a Jew."

"The countess then backtracked. She said I was a mystery and remarkable and wants to know more of me before advising you. We plan to lunch together in the next few weeks. I don't know what she expects from me."

"Act as you always do, confidant and truthful, no matter what" Andrew said immediately. "She hates a liar and can spot one from miles away."

Rachel sighed. "I've seen her powers already but I'm going to forget the countess for now., This has been a most magical week. This trip has meant the world to me. Thank you."

"It takes an odd duck to love an odd duck," Andrew said.

"Indeed it does," Rachel said, taking advantage of a pause in the music, began to rise on her tiptoes to kiss Andrew's cheek.

Andrew held her down by the waist. "Not here. Too many eyes. We've time enough...Speaking of odd ducks, where the devil has Ol' Tom got to tonight?"

Rachel laughed. "Ol' Tom wouldn't be comfortable here for even a second. He's rounding on the pubs to collect bets he and I made on the *Glory B.* He said the odds were too good not to lay some money down. I expect we've made more than the prize pot itself."

Andrew could only shake his head at the girl in his arms who defied all expectations. Rachel, exuberant, danced next with each of her five dragoon shipmates.

When the ball finally ended, Andrew escorted Rachel back to the Canute Castle Hotel. Reaching the third floor, Rachel knocked on Ol' Tom's door but no one answered.

"I knew he'd be out collecting bets and getting soused," Rachel surmised. "I doubt he'll be back until daybreak."

"Must I leave you now?" Andrew said.

"No. At the least, I'll need help getting out of this gown."

"Who helped you into it?" Andrew asked.

"Ol' Tom. He had returned to the hotel for a moment to change clothes and aided me."

"Now I'm jealous."

"He's the one who forced my father to get me off the ship," Rachel said, opening the door to her room. "Ol' Tom was more worried than father that I couldn't be protected after a couple of close calls."

"Were you afraid?" Andrew asked, following her in.

Rachel paused. "Yes, of course. But I never let on to my father or Ol' Tom. I couldn't show weakness if I wanted to remain on board."

In a rush of feeling, Andrew kissed her hand.

"I don't want to hear of the close calls, he said. "They would make me sad and angry."

Rachel shut the door and secured the slide bolt. Only a candle near the door provided light. She then pulled Andrew close and kissed him on the lips. "I've wanted to do this all evening. I suppose you oughtn't be here. I've never invited a man to my room. In truth, I've never had a room to invite anyone to. But this has been the best weekend of my life and I don't want it to end."

"The dragoons who helped crew the boat believe me to be the luckiest man alive," Andrew said. "They're all in awe of you, as I have been from the second we met."

"All those years at sea, I had no friends my age, girl or boy," Rachel said. "I'm not sure what it means to be in love, but I know I want to spend every minute possible with you."

"I feel the same."

"You do?

"I do."

The young couple embraced again.

"When the Countess told me she wanted you to discard me like a broken pipe, I almost fainted," Rachel whispered. "What will you do if she doesn't approve of me?"

Andrew's brow furrowed in the dark, lit only by the

candle and the moonlight from the window. "My feelings for you will not change, but we need her and my brother on our side."

Rachel nodded toward a lamp, which Andrew lit with a match.

"Perhaps," she said, sighing as she sat on a chair beside the bed, "You might unlace my boots? With all these petticoats, I can't see my feet."

Andrew knelt, then unlaced and removed each boot.

"Thank you," Rachel said as she stood and kissed him again. "Now unlace my dress in the back."

"Are you sure about this?"

"Absolutely. Look at it. I can't sleep in this suit of armor."

Rachel turned, allowing Andrew to kiss the back of her bare neck.

"That feels good," she purred. "These days I rather like being a girl and nurse, but I can't help but wonder why people create such monstrosities as these gowns?"

Andrew laughed. "I've not a clue."

He fell silent as he slowly unlaced her dress. It dropped to the floor and she stepped out of it. She started to drop the first of the ten petticoats too but Andrew seized her hands.

"Let me," he murmured. "I want to remove anything you'll allow me to."

Andrew trembled as he removed the petticoats one by one, revealing a camisole hidden under a corset that went from her chest to her tightly cinched waist.

"Now unlace this bloody corset," Rachel breathed.

"You're sure?"

"It is worse than shackles."

Andrew laughed.

"Ol' Tom actually got you into these contraptions?"

"I had no one else. He bound my chest before the race."

When the corset fell away, she was left in the camisole only, breathing deeply. Still facing away, she crossed her arms over her chest. Closing her eyes, she hesitated, dropped her arms, turned to Andrew, and kissed him once again.

"What now?" she asked. "I'm in foreign waters with no compass or chart. I need you to guide me."

"What do you know?" Andrew asked. "You're a nurse, so I expect some knowledge."

"I know only some about how this works, I fear. When ashore in most ports, the sailors, even Ol' Tom and my father, went to brothels or found women in the pubs. They would lie about what they were doing. But I figured it out. I was led to believe it was quite a normal thing to do. It seemed they returned in short order with smiles on their faces. I can't imagine the women were as pleased, for they often appeared only a moment later, looking for other customers. To them it was a business and nothing more."

"Strange that you could fix a dislocated finger with the confidence of Julius Caeser," Andrew said, "yet know nothing of this."

"It seems that my father, Ol' Tom, my tutor, Miss Brown, and now my aunt made sure of it. From the novels I've read, there must be more. Is it only that I care for you?"

"No," Andrew said, "it's that we care for each other. I will put a smile on both our faces."

"What then do I do?" Rachel asked.

Andrew smiled at her innocence. "Start with the buttons on my tunic whilst I feast my eyes upon you."

"Isn't that a waste of time? You can do it so much quicker."

"Not at all. Anticipation of what lies ahead is key," Andrew said. "We've all night and a bit of the morning. Even if Ol' Tom pounds on the door, we'll not answer."

Rachel smiled as she started on the top brass button of the dress uniform of the King's Dragoons Guards. "I will kiss you with every piece I remove."

Soon they stood facing each other in flimsy

undergarments that hid nothing.

"You were correct," Rachel murmured, rubbing her stomach, "the slow tempo has created a delightful ache." Rachel tried but couldn't avoid looking downward. "It appears large," she mumbled.

Andrew smiled and said, "God must have used every trick in his book to create a woman as exquisite as you."

Rachel shivered and pulled the camisole over her head, dropping it to the floor on top of the pile of discarded clothing. Andrew filled his lungs then exhaled through pursed lips. She backed slowly toward the bed. Andrew, already erect, followed.

As they laid side by side, face to face, Rachel began to breathe rapidly.

"Slow," Andrew said, touching his index finger to her lips. "I'm going to explore every inch of you with my eyes and lips. It will take a while. But it will be my fingers and tongue that will take you to places you can't imagine. Places you and I will visit again and again."

He started on her forehead, then eyelids, ears, mouth and neck. Slow and deliberate, with soft lips and a caressing tongue. When he reached her neck with his lips, his fingers gently twirled her nipples until they hardened. Her breathing became rapid again and he whispered, "Slow."

As he explored her breasts with this tongue, he massaged her stomach and slowly moved downward between her legs.

She began to purr with a low guttural whisper through closed lips. "I can't help it," she cried.

He did not stop her, knowing she couldn't. He moved between her legs and explored her thighs with his lips, right then left and back, each time higher, until he separated her lips with his tongue and let his fingers explore her depths.

"Don't stop," Rachel whispered. She began to move rhythmically against his vibrating tongue, wanting more. "Don't stop." She grabbed his head and forced his tongue deeper against her excitement until her body shook and the purring morphed into guttural moans of pleasure.

"Oh my God," she cried, falling back against the pillow. "I didn't know such pleasure existed. Thank you. I am yours."

Rachel knew more was to come. She bent her knees and opened her legs as he rose atop her. Propped on his hands, Andrew and leaned forward to kiss her for the thousandth time.

"Is it going to hurt?" Rachel asked.

"Only for a few heartbeats," Andrew said. "Then never again."

She reached for his firmness and whispered, "Is it too big for me?" Not waiting or caring for an answer, she guided him in.

Together they met resistance but moved together in cadence, each time a bit deeper, until all resistance faded and he entered her depths.

He pulled back and went deeper yet and now the guttural sounds belonged to both of them. As he went deeper, she put her hands on his buttocks and pulled him to the bottom.

"I love you," Andrew said, then emitted a low-pitched guttural sound as he released all his love and collapsed onto her chest.

Now softened, he propped himself up, her face mere inches away.

"That was intense," he said. "I've never felt so satisfied and happy." He then rolled to the side and put his head on her shoulder.

"We are one," Rachel said, still breathing heavily. "The novels of love I've read now make sense to me. It felt good to have you inside me, joined and connected. It's as if there was no way to tell where I end and you begin."

They curled in a ball with his arm around her shoulder, his hand cupping a breast. Her hand covered his hand. He nibbled on the nape of her neck softly and she started to purr once again.

"This truly was the best day ever," Rachel said.

"Yes, it was," Andrew agreed. "Tell me, did you study Shakespeare all those years at sea?"

"No. Why? My tutor, Goose, uh, Miss Brown, read some to me. It seemed Mr. Shakespeare kept killing people off with little reason."

"Yes, I suppose he did. But did your Goose not read Shakespeare's thoughts on love?"

Rachel laughed. "She's not my goose, that's her nickname. But not that I recall." Rachel nestled close to Andrew. "Recite some."

"I believe Romeo and Juliet is his best," Andrew opined.

"I stopped listening to Goose when she told me both of them die at the end."

"True, but the things they said earlier are beautiful." He cleared his throat. "*My bounty is as boundless as the sea, my love as deep. The more I give to thee, the more I have, for both are infinite.*"

"That is beautiful," Rachel said.

"When Romeo first sees Juliet, he falls in love straightaway. '*O, she doth teach the torches to burn bright! It seems she hangs upon the cheek of night like a rich jewel in an Ethiope's ear; beauty too rich for use, for earth too dear*!"

Rachel started to giggle.

"What's so funny? It's beautiful," Andrew said.

"It t'is, but when I first saw you, I thought you an insufferable fool, complaining about nothing. Besides, I've been to Ethiopia. They're a sorry lot."

"What changed?"

"You trusted me to fix your finger," Rachel said, still giggling, "and then asked for a formal introduction. The perfect gentleman."

"I wish I had more to offer you at the moment," Andrew said. "I would marry you in the morning if I didn't think we'd incur the wrath of my family and yours."

"If there's a question in there," Rachel said, "the answer is yes." Rachel kissed Andrew on the lips, then rolled back and brought Andrew's hand atop her breast again, holding it there. "A most definite yes."

They awoke at 9 a.m. with the morning sun baking the room.

"Last night, in the heat of things," Rachel said tentatively, "you asked me to marry you. Were you serious?"

"I was. Would you like me to ask again?"

Rachel nodded. "Yes. I liked the sound of it."

Andrew, still naked, got off the bed, walked around to the other side, and knelt next to Rachel, who was lying on her side but having a difficult time not laughing. He took her hands in his.

"Rachel, the word love had no meaning until I met you. It would be impossible for this poor army officer to love you more than I do now. But I know that tomorrow and each day thereafter, I will love you even more."

As Andrew spoke, Rachel could see tears forming in each of his eyes.

"Will you marry me and make me the happiest man in the world? I want us to share every thought, good or bad, and every secret."

Rachel nodded, whispering "Yes to all of it," as the tears welled up in her eyes as well.

They made love once again.

Afterward, as they lay exhausted, nose to nose, Rachel whispered, "Do you think we might be allowed to live in this bed for the rest of our lives? I would consider it."

Andrew laughed and got out of bed, seeing an envelope slid under the door jamb.

"It's from Ol' Tom," he said. He opened the envelope and removed a wad of bills and a note. He counted the money first. “There’s fifty-five pounds here. Pretty decent for a five-pound wager. A shame you hadn’t bet more.” He handed the note to Rachel which she opened and read aloud.

> *My dear Ray,*
> *I took the morning train back to Bournemouth. Didn’t want to wake you. Here’s your winnings. Quite the day.*
> *I’ll give my love from you to Betty Baugh and Little Tom. I expect word of our victory will have already found its way to Bournemouth. It’ll keep the stories going for a year. I’ll never swear that you or I were there.*
> *Don't let what's for you go by you. You belong with Andrew. He loves you. The Captain would have loved him too. Until our sails cross again.*
> *Ol’ Tom*

Rachel smiled. “I guess Ol’ Tom got there before you did.”

After bathing and dressing in travel clothes, Andrew and Rachel went downstairs for a late breakfast.

“Do we tell your aunt and uncle of our engagement?” Andrew asked.

“I think they’ll figure it out quick enough,” Rachel said. “Aunt Cynthia for sure.”

“Next you have to win over Olivia,” Andrew said. “We’ll need her support and my brother’s wealth at some point.”

“She can’t stop me from loving you.”

“Nor I for you. But an army life is hard on a marriage. I have four months left on this enlistment and I will need to re-enlist for at least another three years. If so, I will likely be gone for long periods and in some jeopardy. I would be miserable being away from you. But

I need to be in the army long enough to earn a generous pension. Absent that, I won't have the funds to support us and a family."

Rachel smiled and reached across the table to hold Andrew's hands. "All my days and nights 'til now will be but a memory. I've a new life now with you in it. Finish your current duty and obligations in the army and we'll be fine. We don't need anyone's approval, including your brother, Olivia, or my aunt and uncle."

"How so? I've no inheritance," Andrew asked.

"Have we now sworn no secrets between us?" Rachel asked.

"Yes, we did."

"Then I need to disclose something," she said. "A thing my uncle made me swear to tell no one."

"But you're going to tell me?" Andrew asked.

"I need to."

"And that is?"

"I'm richer than the Lydian king, Croesus, on my own from my father's estate," Rachel said. "According to Uncle Simon, I'm richer than him. This is a secret and you must not tell anyone, including your brother or the countess. Let them believe we're poor. I promised to tell Simon and Cynthia before disclosing it to anyone else."

Andrew sat back in his chair and shook his head in disbelief.

"I promise."

"I've made my choice. You finish your current enlistment – four months and no more. And then we build a life together."

On the Monday train back to London, Rachel and Andrew tried to figure out the best way to break the news to her aunt and uncle.

"I haven't the faintest idea how to tell them," Rachel said. "They're not that different from Olivia. They've said they like you and they know you've made me happy. Then they turn around and say they have men for me to meet who are Jewish."

Andrew said, "I'd like not to alienate either family. Whatever we do, wherever we go, my brother and Olivia have connections. They can still be helpful. We don't want to be on their bad side."

"And I want to continue learning medicine from Simon and Cynthia," Rachel said. "They are my only family and as close to parents as I'll ever have. I know they love me and I love them. I can't hurt them."

"Why does love have to be so complicated?" Andrew moaned, laying his head on Rachel's shoulder.

"Do you think Simon and Cynthia will suspect we've been intimate?"

"If they ask, you'll deny it and they'll accept it, then when alone they'll question it. I would," Andrew said.

"Perhaps we should wait until I've met with Olivia. That's half the battle."

As the train pulled into the Salisbury station outside London, Rachel and Andrew remained unsure how to go about telling their families of their engagement. They did agree that they would break the news to both families after Rachel's luncheon with Olivia, whether that meeting went well or not. Only then would they deal with the consequences.

Chapter Ten
Andrew

Rachel and Andrew's cab stopped at the front door of the Romain house just after two p.m.

"You best not come in," Rachel said. "They'll see how we look at each other and know we did more than race a boat this week."

"I won't argue," Andrew said. "But I will be sad the moment I leave you." He deposited Rachel's valise at the front door and climbed back into the cab.

Simon had left for the hospital early in the morning but returned before noon, cancelling his afternoon appointments in order to receive Rachel at home, along with Cynthia.

As soon as Rachel entered the door, she yelled, "I'm home!" Sharron appeared first, followed by Cynthia, then Simon.

"You're back and in one piece," Cynthia fussed. "We were worried, of course. I made Simon cancel much of his Monday office."

Rachel said, "So much to tell." Smiling, she hugged Cynthia, Sharron, and Simon in turn.

"This morning's London Times," Simon said, holding up a folded newspaper, "reported that Captain Andrew Drayer of the First King's Dragoon Guards and five fellow dragoons won the Cowes Week Regatta. The Royal Army is celebrating everywhere, whilst the Royal Navy dismisses the victory as balderdash. The Royal Navy spokesman claims the dragoons were merely helpers and the sloop, the *Glory B*, was captained by a mysterious former Royal Navy admiral in disguise and his young lieutenant."

"I don't know where to start," Rachel said, laughing. "Let's all sit for lunch. I'll begin with our search in Bournemouth for my father's retired first mate, Ol' Tom Voz. Afterward, I must write him to say he's been elevated to admiral."

Simon, Cynthia and Sharron listened raptly for two hours as Rachel divulged her weekend's escapade in detail.

"This morning," Rachel lied, concluding her tale. "Andrew left the Royal Navy barracks, picked me up at the hotel, and we boarded the train to come home."

"What an adventure," Cynthia said. "It's the stuff of fairytales!"

Simon added, "And I assume Captain Drayer and his dragoon friends were perfect gentlemen the entire time?"

"No, not at all," Rachel said. 'Most gentlemen I've met in England do as they please, with little care for the people around them. Andrew and his men were quite the opposite, I'd say."

Rachel's audience of three raised eyebrows until she added, "Tis I that was the gentleman and they the peons and servants. Ol' Tom and I yelled ourselves hoarse giving orders constantly to all of them, including Andrew. Wonderous, indeed, that they all listened, obeyed, and said 'Aye, Aye, Captain.'"

Sharron started laughing, followed by Cynthia, then Simon.

Soon, Simon regretfully announced that he needed to return to the office to see patients. Cynthia asked Rachel to join her in the parlor.

"How do you see your relationship with Andrew?" Cynthia asked once they were alone.

"This is all so new to me," Rachel said. "I thoroughly enjoy Andrew's company. You must know how much I appreciate him for planning this adventure. I don't believe any other man would have."

"But you must understand the difficulties with Andrew going forward. I do think you should broaden your horizons with other men with whom there is more compatibility."

"There is but one incompatibility," Rachel countered, her face as stubbornly stony as it was the day she arrived at the Romain door.

“But it is a significant one for our family and his,” Cynthia said gently.

“Perhaps,” Rachel said, “but for now I would like to bask in the glow of the past weekend. The last two gentlemen you introduced me to didn’t even believe that I lived on a ship, and thought my desire to become a working nurse ridiculous. They thought you being a nurse made no sense as well. Andrew encourages me at every step.”

Cynthia paused. “Little do they know. I’ll admit,” she said, “that Andrew’s a rare fellow.”

Rachel beamed and embraced her aunt.

“Everything will be alright,” she said. “You’ll see.”

The next morning at 6 a.m., Cynthia, Simon and Rachel left for the hospital together as usual.

Two days later, Rachel found a letter from Olivia waiting in the entryway. She opened it immediately. Their luncheon was to take place at Brown’s Hotel on Albemarle Street that coming Monday at noon. Rachel responded to Olivia and also sent a note to the dragoon barracks, telling Andrew that the date of the meeting had been set.

That night at dinner, Simon scratched his beard and offered his niece some advice.

“You must listen carefully to what the countess says and say little in return. She comes from a powerful family, and her husband sits in the House of Lords. The earl is held in very high esteem for re-establishing his earldom. You don’t need those kinds of enemies.”

Rachel replied, “I appreciate your input but before I even thought of a strategy, Andrew told me how to act.”

“And that’s how?” Simon asked.

“Be myself. Olivia knows where I’ve been and how I was raised. She figured out I was Ray during the race.”

“She knew you were on the boat? I thought that was a secret?” Simon asked.

“She looked at my wind-blown complexion and

figured it out straightaway," Rachel said. "If I act the shy, demure girl with no thoughts, she'll know it's an act. I will say what I feel and think. That should carry me home."

"I hope you know what you're doing," Cynthia said, her face betraying a worried expression. "Royalty in England barely tolerate Jews. You cannot ruffle too many feathers. Be careful."

Rachel arrived at Brown's Hotel fifteen minutes early. She introduced herself to the maître d' and told him she would wait in the ornate hotel lobby for the countess. At ten past noon, a waiter escorted Rachel to Olivia's table, placed discreetly in the rear corner of the room. Rachel performed a slight curtsy and Olivia extended her hand toward a chair.

After a few pleasantries, Olivia again thanked Rachel for the victory in the Cowes Week Regatta. A waiter came and was shooed away by Olivia. "We've things to discuss."

Olivia turned her attention back to Rachel. "Your victory has caused a bit of a pickle," Olivia said, albeit with a sly smile.

"I'm sorry," Rachel said. "I hope not too serious."

Olivia laughed. "It will pass. The Royal Navy and some of our yacht club members are put out because we used Royal Army men to take the cup. Our victory made them look incompetent. Funny actually. They are desperate to know the name of our captain whom they believe was a Royal Navy admiral in disguise. I told them he said his name is Tom and that's all I could recall."

Rachel laughed, put at ease by Olivia's easy manner. "Tom it is," Rachel said. "He was a cabin boy on the HMS Victory at Trafalgar. He saw Lord Nelson get shot by a French musketeer and ran to get the ship surgeon."

"I'm glad to know but let's keep Tom's identity between us, shall we? I'll cut to the chase, my dear. What are your intentions with my poor brother-in-law?"

Olivia asked. “He seems quite overmatched by your presence.”

“I assure you he is not,” Rachel said, “except aboard a ship.”

“Or in a surgeon’s office.”

“Yes, that too.”

“He is quite captivated by you. As are his friends in the King’s Guard. I asked them.”

Rachel laughed. “Andrew told me Kenneth and Sam were jealous.”

“All of them are jealous. I don’t see how this can go anywhere without ending badly,” Olivia opined. “You’re a Jewess who works as a nurse. He is a penniless Captain without a pension unless he becomes a career soldier. The Earl purchased the cash bond for Andrew’s commission as a captain and bought his uniforms and horse. Not to mention his schooling prior to enlisting.”

“Thank you for that,” Rachel said, the smile having vanished from her face, wondering if the earl and Olivia expected to be repaid for the kindnesses they had offered to Andrew. If so, she’d settle Andrew’s score.

“I’m sorry my dear, but my husband and I see no point in you continuing your pursuit of Andrew,” Olivia said.

“I believe you’ve got that backward. Andrew has pursued me,” Rachel said defiantly. “My aunt, uncle and I are surprised each time he calls.”

“Then what could you have given him to keep him in your grip? I don’t understand, unless you are offering sexual favors.”

Rachel knew decorum and Olivia had crossed that line. Rachel stood, not averting her eyes from Olivia. “Your Ladyship offends me with that accusation. I am a virgin and will remain one until I marry,” Rachel lied, her gaze straight at Olivia. “Should I take leave or will you offer an apology?”

Olivia’s face turned bright red as she realized she couldn’t intimidate Rachel. After a long and uncomfortable pause, Olivia said, "Please accept my apology. My comment was uncalled for."

Rachel sat again. "Thank you."

Still blushing, Olivia remained silent until Rachel spoke again.

"Let's say, for argument's sake, that I did marry Andrew. I've been to Calcutta and Bombay and I've seen how the lower castes are regarded. Would you and the earl treat Andrew as an undesirable?"

"He'd be destitute."

"If Andrew found gainful employment and was no burden on the family, would he and I be welcome at your manor for Christmas dinner, at the wedding of his nephews and niece, or on the *Glory B?"*

"I see your years on the ship has made you tough. You get straight to the point and I like that," Olivia said. "At the ball in Southampton, I called you remarkable. I meant it. You're not like most Jews, who crumble when threatened."

Rachel ignored this backhanded compliment and pressed the issue.

"You didn't answer my question. Would we be welcome in your manor?"

Olivia sighed heavily. "Yes. I'm very fond of Andrew and I suppose I always will be."

"And the earl? Would he welcome us and our children?"

"He'll do what I say," Olivia said. "As long as Andrew's not an embarrassment or a drain on our finances."

"Good," Rachel said. "Then you'll be welcome at my house as well. Just so you know, if Andrew asks me to marry, I don't know how I could say no."

Olivia laughed. "Yes, by God, you do have spunk. Shall we order lunch and you'll tell me of your years at sea?"

Olivia raised her hand and the waiter reappeared in a second. After the long lunch and sharing of stories on each side, Olivia said, "I must get going. This has been most enjoyable. I must say, I look forward to seeing you again. I never thought I'd welcome a Jew into our family, but if Andrew chooses you, so be it. I'll not stand in his way, nor will the earl."

Rachel countered with, "It's not like I or my aunt and uncle ever imagined having an earl and countess on my wedding guest list. But here we are. I've enjoyed spending time with you as well."

Andrew appeared at the Romain's house after dinner that night, to take Rachel for an evening stroll and find out how the meeting with Olivia went. Rachel told Andrew everything, including the part about offering sexual favors and how she responded.

"Olivia knows nothing of my trust fund," Rachel said. "Still, she said that if we married and you and I were not financial burdens, then we'd be welcome for Christmas dinner. You were correct that I needed to hold my own. At the ball and today, Olivia described me as remarkable and said she looked forward to seeing me again. Those exact words."

Andrew shook his head in disbelief. "I don't know how I could possibly love you more, but I do. Now to work on Simon and Cynthia."

"That may pose the greater challenge," Rachel conceded.

"When we marry, not if," Andrew said. "I know what I'll do for employment."

"Tell me?"

"I'll start reading legal texts and apprentice with a barrister," Andrew said. "My second cousin, Burt Drayer, is a barrister. He's the son of my grand-uncle. He apprenticed with Sir William Blackstone, who is considering starting a school of law at Oxford. Burt and I have always gotten along, and I'm sure he'll take me on or find someone who will."

Rachel beamed. "A delightful idea. Can one make a

good living at the law?"

"If I'm good, very much so," Andrew proclaimed.

"Then you must be good," she said. "For now, because of my promise to Simon and Cynthia, you must pretend to believe I am as poor as a church mouse when you ask +for my hand. You'll come to dinner this Sunday. When we sit in the parlor, you'll ask to speak to my aunt and uncle alone."

Andrew laughed. "Aye, Aye, Captain. I always thought charging through enemy cannon fire at a gallop would be difficult, but this ..."

Circling back to the house, Andrew said his goodbyes to the Romains, leaving Rachel in the parlor with Cynthia

"I must admit," Cynthia said, putting aside her embroidery, "you've been glowing ever since you returned from Southampton. It's nice to see."

"He makes me so happy," Rachel gushed. Then she repeated what she had told Olivia. "If Andrew does ask me to marry, I don't know how I could say no."

Cynthia shook her head.

That night, Cynthia told Simon of her conversation with Rachel. "Rachel is in love, and I fear Andrew will propose soon. What shall we do?"

"I've never seen her happier," Simon said. "Andrew does go out of his way to see to it and supports everything she does and how she acts. None of the suitors we've found will accept that."

"Do you think Andrew knows of her trust fund?"

"Rachel swears he knows nothing of her moneys. If we deny them, I believe she'll leave our house and marry anyway. If he asks, we must say we'll welcome him gladly, as difficult as that may be."

"Knowing Rachel, do you think this past weekend had only to do with boating?" Cynthia asked.

"Does it matter what I believe," Simon said.

Cynthia's shoulders sagged as she mused, "The

thought of hosting the Earl and Countess Brandler, among others, is ..."

"Say no more," Simon interrupted. "I've been thinking of that for a while. Too much to contemplate."

The following Sunday, Andrew posed the question to Simon and Cynthia. When both said they'd happily comply with whatever Rachel desired, Andrew ran out of the parlor, took a knee, and placed a simple band on Rachel's finger. Rachel, in turn, ran into the parlor with tears of joy and gave her aunt and uncle hugs, kisses and thank-yous.

The following week, Andrew told the countess and the earl, who had already assumed the worst and were not surprised.

As Andrew would not convert to Judaism and Rachel had no desire to be a member of the Church of England, they decided on a civil marriage with little fanfare and a small celebration with only Cynthia, Simon and Andrew's closest friends. Not surprisingly, the countess and the earl begged off. Cynthia and Rachel went shopping for a simple wedding dress and booked a small restaurant nearby for the party. The wedding would take place six weeks hence on a Saturday afternoon.

Everything fell into place. Andrew secured his law apprenticeship with his cousin, Burt Drayer, and his commission in the British Army was set to end on October first. The married couple would live with Simon and Cynthia after Andrew's commission expired. Only then would Simon allow Rachel to tell Andrew of her trust fund.

Two weeks later, a month before the wedding, Rachel, ebullient, sat at the dinner table with Simon and Cynthia when a loud knock on the door startled them.

"I'll get it," Sharron said, poking her head in.

"No, I'll do it. I'm certain it's Andrew," Rachel said. "He was instructing new recruits. Perhaps he can stay for dinner."

She ran to the door only to find Kenneth Eakes and Sam McCollum wearing dirty officer uniforms. Both had streaks of blood on their shirts. Both held their heads low as they entered the foyer. Rachel gripped the doorframe, knowing something was amiss with Andrew.

Sam mumbled, "We're so sorry."

"What has happened? Where is Andrew?" Rachel screamed.

The men shook their heads, their eyes bloodshot from crying but unable to speak.

Where is he? Damn you, tell me!"

Kenneth spoke haltingly, unable to look Rachel in the eye. "He was thrown from his horse during training."

"Take me to him," Rachel cried. "My uncle will come too. Simon, hurry! Andrew is hurt!"

"It's too late, Rachel," Sam whispered. "It's too late. Andrew is dead."

"No!" Rachel wailed. "It can't be! Please God, no."

Rachel extended her hands out as if shoving the men away and started walking backward, away from the source of her grief. Her eyes rolled, then her hand shot out blindly to the side, looking for support. Simon and Cynthia arrived in the foyer in time to catch a sobbing Rachel as she collapsed.

"What did you tell her?" Simon demanded. "What of Andrew?"

"Andrew was thrown from his horse and killed, sir," Sam said.

"Oh, what terrible news," Cynthia gasped.

"Help me lift her and take her up to her room," Simon ordered the two dragoons.

Kenneth and Sam carried Rachel to her bedroom with Sharron, Cynthia and Simon following close behind. After laying Rachel atop her bed, Simon pulled the two dragoons into the hallway and down the stairs to the foyer.

"What happened, in detail?" he asked.

"It was a routine training session with new recruits on the fields north of the barracks," Sam said. "Andrew was leading twenty recruits in a coordinated charge with standard lances. He rode his favorite horse; it's one he's ridden for over a year. Andrew looked back to see how the men were doing as we went from muddy to firm ground. The quick shift in weight and the change in the ground caused the horse to lose its balance. Andrew and the horse tumbled forward."

Sam paused, his face pale, looking to his friend to take over.

Kenneth continued. "Andrew hit the ground head first and landed ahead of his horse. The men behind him couldn't stop and two horses rode atop him. Four horses stumbled and one dragoon fractured his leg, another his arm. Andrew's horse's left front leg was shattered and was put down."

"A black day if ever there was one," Sam swore.

"What happens now?" Simon asked.

"His next of kin are being notified," Kenneth said. "They will make funeral arrangements."

"There will be a full inquiry, I expect," Sam cut in hastily. "It's our first training death in eleven years."

Simon put both hands to his face then looked up. "Rachel has never been happier. I don't know how long she will mourn."

"Andrew told us of the engagement and we had planned a party to celebrate," Kenneth said. "To a man, ever since the boating victory on the Solent, our brigade thought Andrew to be the luckiest man on earth."

"The colonel gave us leave to tell Rachel," Sam said. "We have to get back. One of us will return as soon as we know the funeral arrangements."

With that, Andrew's best friends bowed their heads, turned and headed back to where their horses waited in the street.

The next morning at breakfast, neither Simon nor Cynthia had much appetite. Rachel had not come down, nor touched the tray outside her room.

'Remember how it was when Jacob left her here?" Simon said softly. "I thought that was bad, but at least she knew deep down that she couldn't go back to sea. Now, all the joy in her life has been snuffed out."

"What should we do?" Cynthia asked.

"Nothing to do, I fear. We wait. When she's ready to work again, we can only hope it will occupy her mind, body and spirit."

"If Andrew were Jewish," Cynthia said, "he'd be buried today. I have no idea what his family will do or when the funeral will take place. It bothers me."

"We've no control," Simon said. "Probably his brother's vast estate has its own cemetery."

Cynthia nodded agreement. "I would think the Earl would have a bishop to do the service. I'm not sure we'll be welcome."

"Please," Simon said, his face growing hard. "They were engaged. Of course we'll be welcome."

All day and the next one too, food and drink deposited outside Rachel's door continued to sit largely untouched. On the second night, Rachel appeared at dinner but kept her head down and refused to speak. She returned to her room after finishing only a portion of the meal.

After dinner, Sharron answered a knock on the front door, then came to the dining room.

"The Countess Brandler to see Rachel," Sharron announced.

Simon and Cynthia went to the foyer, introduced themselves to Olivia, then escorted her into the parlor.

Once seated, Olivia asked, "How is Rachel doing, or do I need ask?"

"She's been crying in her room for two days and nights," Cynthia said.

"I've come personally," Olivia said, "because we have an issue with Andrew's funeral. I've only a short time."

"Do we need to get Rachel?" Simon asked.

"No. What I have to say would only upset her more," Olivia answered.

Simon and Cynthia exchanged glances.

"What is the issue?" Cynthia asked.

"We were obliged to tell our bishop about Andrew's intention to marry a Jew, and he was furious. He met with Andrew the following night and forbade him from marrying Rachel. Andrew told the bishop to go straight to hell."

"Oh my," Cynthia said. "That couldn't have been well received."

"It was not, and when we told the bishop of Andrew's death, he told us ..." Olivia paused, struggling to get the words out. "He told us it was God's punishment."

"Monstrous," Simon said with feeling.

"I quite agree," Olivia said, her eyes full of tears. "Realize, the funeral must be held at our estate in the family's sanctuary and Andrew will be buried in the family cemetery. The bishop has forbidden us to invite Rachel or you."

The parlor became quiet until Olivia spoke again. "The earl and I argued against his decision, but the bishop was unrelenting. Our hands are tied."

"It's so cruel to Rachel," Cynthia said quietly.

"Andrew's company of dragoons happen to agree. They were asked to be the pallbearers. When they discovered Rachel would not be allowed to attend the funeral, they refused to attend.

"They all knew Rachel from the cricket matches and the Cowes Regatta," Simon said.

"And they adored her," Olivia added.

"What now?" Cynthia asked.

"Their commanding officer, Colonel Newman, arrived at a solution which I hope is acceptable. Two services. One which will take place first, at the King's Guard chapel on Friday at 2 p.m., led by the Guard's deacon. Our bishop will not know of it. From there, the hearse will take Andrew's casket to our estate for the second service and the burial. My secretary will send the details by tomorrow eve."

"Should we tell Rachel the whole story?" Simon asked.

"If you wish. She'd find out soon enough," Olivia said.

"I'm not sure how much more distress Rachel can handle," Cynthia said.

"From what little I know of Rachel, she is strong, resilient, and has seen death before. I believe, given time, she'll be able to ... move on."

"We hope so," Simon said, taking Cynthia's hand in his.

Cynthia entered Rachel's room after a soft knock. Rachel lay supine on her bed, staring at the ceiling.

"Olivia was here. She came to invite us to the funeral," Cynthia said. "It will be at the chapel at the King's Guard barracks, Friday at two."

Rachel blinked, then sat up. "Not at the family estate?"

Cynthia sat gently on the side of the bed.

"Their bishop would not allow Jews to attend. He was against the marriage. In fact, he met with Andrew after the announcement to dissuade him. Apparently, Andrew told him to go to hell."

Rachel smiled for the first time in days. "He would say that. I would have told a rabbi the same."

"Let's hope you never have to do that," Cynthia responded. "A service at the estate will follow the one at the barracks. Colonel Newman and the dragoons insisted on a funeral where you'd be welcome."

Rachel's eyes filled with tears as she laid back down.

"I'll tailor black dresses with muted crepe for you and me."

Rachel agreed with a nod. Cynthia waited, motionless, until Rachel spoke.

"Why has God abandoned me?" Rachel whispered.

"God would never abandon you, my darling," Cynthia said, reaching out to stroke Rachel's face.

"He has," cried Rachel hoarsely. "My own father abandoned me, and I lost the only life I'd ever known. I lost my mother before I knew her. Then I lost my father in a typhoon half way around the world. When I found someone to truly love, he dies. I feel so damn abandoned."

Rachel began to sob.

"You're not abandoned," Cynthia whispered. "Simon and I love you and we are here for you every day."

Rachel nodded, moved over and patted the bed, inviting Cynthia to lie next to her, Cynthia laid down next to her and hugged her."

"My first husband died when I was nineteen," Cynthia said. "I thought my life was over. I believed I would be a spinster until I died. Then I met Simon, and it was like my life began again. We wanted a family so badly, but I miscarried time after time. I thought God had abandoned me too. But then I received the best gift and I've been happy ever since."

Rachel's head picked off the bed. "Gift?"

"You," Cynthia said. "You gave me the chance to be a mother and I've loved every second of it. Even the challenges, of which there have been many."

Rachel rolled her head onto Cynthia's shoulder and began to cry.

"I was ... so in love," Rachel said between sobs. "I was so excited ... for the future ... with Andrew. I don't think ... I can ever ... find that again."

"You may or you may not, but know that Simon and I will stay by you."

Cynthia, now crying, kissed Rachel on the cheek.

"I don't remember my mother at all. Could I call you Mum?" Rachel asked.

Cynthia embraced Rachel. "I'd like nothing more."

After clearing the guard gate, the cab delivered the Romains to the chapel on the army base. Outside the chapel, Kenneth, Sam, and the other dragoons from Andrew's regiment stood awaiting Rachel's arrival.

Andrew's fellow officers aided Simon and Cynthia out of the cab. Then Kenneth and Sam helped Rachel down and escorted her, arm in arm, into the chapel. Another dragoon took Cynthia's arm and asked Simon to follow.

The group walked to the front of the sanctuary where three chairs had been reserved. Before sitting, Sam and Kenneth escorted Rachel to the open casket, which was surrounded by flowers. Andrew, dressed in his King's Guard dress uniform, lay in quiet repose, his face betraying no evidence of his violent end. Rachel, already weeping, fell into Kenneth's arms; he escorted her back to her seat. Olivia and the earl sat in the chairs next to Rachel and gave what silent comfort they could.

After the service, Olivia introduced her husband, Anthony, the earl, to the Romains. While the earl chatted with Simon and Cynthia, Olivia pulled Rachel aside.

"I'll tell you what I told your aunt and uncle the other night," Olivia said. "I think your years at sea took the spoil out of you. I know you will move past this terrible tragedy and make something special of your life. I had looked forward to having you as a sister-in-law."

"Thank you," Rachel sniffled. "I told Andrew the same about you."

"Hopefully," Olivia added, "we'll meet again in happier times. Perhaps another luncheon."

"I'd like that."

"We must be going," Olivia said. "Can't make that arse of a bishop wait."

Olivia gave Rachel a hug goodbye, then entered her waiting carriage, which followed Andrew's hearse out of the base.

That night at dinner, Rachel, Cynthia and Simon said little. Even Sharron, used to chattering, served the food and disappeared.

At end of the meal, Rachel said, "I'll take this weekend to think of Andrew. He was so proud I wanted to be a surgical nurse. It's already the seventh day of mourning; I need to get back to work."

"Are you sure you're ready?" Simon asked.

"I'm ready," Rachel said. "I need something to distract me."

Simon nodded approvingly but Cynthia shook her head, not in total agreement.

"When I was twelve," Rachel said, "the *Sol Quest* was heading to Madagascar from Calcutta when a violent storm hit. The mainmast collapsed and the rudder snapped. A huge wave pitchpoled[8] the ship, stern over the front. Four seamen were hurled off the deck into the sea, never to be seen again. All we could do was ride out the storm. By morning, the sea was as smooth as glass. The captain said –"

Simon interrupted. "You mean your father?"

"Of course. Anyway, we had too much to repair to mourn the loss of the men. We cut the mainmast away and re-rigged the ship. The helm control of the rudder was useless, so navigation was impossible. Ol' Tom and the men refitted a makeshift rudder below deck. The captain would yell orders to direct the rudder one way or another that I would relay to the men below. For two days, no one slept, but with a bit of luck we made it to Tana safely."

"And here I thought I'd heard all your best stories already," Cynthia marveled. "Were you afraid?"

"That's the point," Rachel said. "We had too much to

---

[8] Pitchpoled: (nautical term) to be overturned so that the boat's stern pitches forward over its bow.

do to be afraid, or to mourn. We had to stay alive. It wasn't until we were secure in port that we spoke of the four men."

"Monday it is then," Simon said. "We've two hernias and an amputation."

Rachel nodded.

Cynthia kept her eyes on Rachel. "You'll have periods of sadness when something reminds you of Andrew."

"Eyes opened or closed, everything will remind me of Andrew," Rachel said.

Chapter Eleven
Semmelweis

Ten days after Andrew's death, Rachel returned to work as a nurse and a student of medicine.

Having become proficient in delivering both ether and chloroform anesthesia, Rachel wanted more.

"I'd like to begin assisting in more complicated surgical procedures," Rachel said. "The anesthesia I find quite boring compared to watching you work."

Simon shook his head. "You are only one of a few hundred in the British Isles who have a gifted hand in delivering anesthetic. It's not easy."

"No, it's not," Rachel said. "But I sit watching the different stages of sleep and nothing else. I want to use my hands."

At first, Simon let Rachel assist with minor surgeries, including hernias and the removal of cysts.

"Wouldn't it be faster if you placed the sutures and I tied them or vice versa?" Rachel asked.

"I suppose," Simon said. "You'd have to learn the knot techniques. You've seen me use various sutures, each with a different purpose - catgut, linen, silk, even hemp."

At night, Simon and Rachel would have knot-tying contests until Simon was no longer winning.

Six months later at the Royal London Hospital, Rachel performed a difficult, incarcerated[9] inguinal hernia operation on an obese firefighter behind locked doors. Simon saw in Rachel's predicament a version of the same prejudice that had impeded his own study of medicine: "One of the great tragedies of living here in England," he said first to Cynthia, and then later to Rachel herself, "or anywhere probably, is that you have hands of gold but cannot get into medical school and

---

[9] Incarcerated hernia: occurs when the contents of the hernia, usually intestine become trapped and cannot be pushed back in.

cannot become a surgeon. There were barriers for me as a Jew, but the ones facing you as a woman are even greater."

Rachel said. "Even if there are places to be trained, I wouldn't be able to work here. I won't leave England. I want to be here with you and mum."

"As time goes on, my dear," Simon said, "and only when possible, I will let you do more and more, just as if you were a surgeon in training."

Cynthia added, "Realize we could all be arrested and Simon would lose his license to practice medicine and surgery if we are discovered."

"Then we must be carcful," Rachel said.

Simon allowed Rachel to perform more and more procedures. At Simon's private clinic with anesthetized patients, discovery was not an issue and Rachel could act as the primary surgeon. At the hospital, Rachel could only operate when Cynthia or another friend of Simon's, a doctor named Dr. Charles Kaplan, gave the anesthetic. Simon would usually wedge a stool next to the closed door. On the rare occasion when another surgeon or nurse would begin to enter the room unannounced, Simon quickly took the reins.

One afternoon after a morning surgery, the knighted, Chairman of the Department of Surgery, Sir Archibald Leach, invited Simon, Cynthia and Rachel to lunch at a café around the corner from the hospital where they were served a thick mutton stew and a dense white bread.

"I have to admit, Simon," Leach said, "your surgical times for procedures is often half of the other surgeons, including me. What's your secret?"

"We work in concert with each other," Simon said, glancing around the table. "My wife and niece know what I'm going to do before I do. I rarely have to ask for an instrument or suture. It's already there."

"Hmmph," Leach said. "Do you think Rachel or

Cynthia would work with the other surgeons?"

"Absolutely not," Cynthia said. "We're busy enough."

Seeing that Leach was a bit put off by Cynthia's quick rejection, Rachel changed the subject.

"May I ask you a question, Sir Archibald?" Rachel asked.

"Of course, my dear," Leach replied.

"Why is it there are no women in medicine or surgery?" Rachel asked.

"Simple answers that are widely known and accepted," Leach said, as he put a hefty piece of mutton in his mouth and talked as he chewed. "As we all know, menstruation makes women unstable and diminishes their reasoning. We can't have surgeons unavailable for a week every month, can we? Besides, the female brain lacks the intellect. It's an affront to nature to let women practice medicine."

"May I respond?" Rachel inquired.

Simon and Cynthia shook their heads, looking apprehensive.

"Besides," Leach continued, ignoring Rachel, "society won't allow women to be exposed to nude men or the blood, guts and morbidity of surgery."

"But we nurses see all that," Rachel replied sharply. "None of that bothers me or Cynthia."

"Bah," Leach said, "Yes, you endure it, but most women wouldn't last a minute. Ought we to teach a hundred women our trade only to find one or two who can finish the course? Of course not. A colossal waste of time and energy. Women are supposed to have children, cook, clean, and run a household. It's God's way."

Cynthia watched Rachel's jaw tighten and teeth bared, like a mad dog ready to pounce. Cynthia grabbed Rachel's forearm and squeezed. Leach, thankfully, was far too interested in dipping his bread into the stew to notice. Rachel shot daggers at Cynthia but got the message and hid her distress.

"What were you thinking?" Simon demanded as they all walked back to their clinic. "One foul word from you and we'd all be barred from using the hospital facilities."

"That man is a horse's arse and a damn fool," Rachel spat.

"Please, Rachel, I had hoped we had purged you of foul language," Simon said with a pained expression.

Cynthia snickered. "My dear, I believe Rachel's diagnosis is quite to the point. Archibald is indeed a horse's arse and a damn fool."

This retort got Rachel laughing. She then hugged Cynthia and whispered, "Thanks, Mum."

Six months later, Simon received notice that Sir Archibald Leach wanted to see him, alone. Knowing of nothing amiss, Simon arrived at Leach's office unprepared for anything but compliments for work well done.

"It's come to my attention," Leach said, "that you may be allowing your niece to perform procedures which she's not, by law, allowed to do. What say you?"

Simon blanched.

"Have – have there been any untoward incidents or complications?"

"No, but that's not the point," Leach said. "If true, you and she are breaking the law and could be punished."

Simon took and deep breath and said stonily, "Rachel Romain is not performing surgery. I am with her every second of every procedure."

Leach studied Simon over the tips of his tented fingers. At last, he said, "I shouldn't have to tell you what will happen to the hospital if the newspapers report that nurses are doing surgical procedures. Even if we refute those claims, the damage is done."

"Tying a knot, cutting suture," Simon said, "or holding an instrument so I can observe is not surgery."

"For God's sake, man, two different sources have

seen her with a scalpel in-hand, making incisions before the scalpel is handed back to you," Leach cried. "It must stop."

Simon, however, could not be stopped. "Are these reports from surgeons who haven't our results or reputation? I put to you that this is a jealous slander."

"It may be so, but if I don't act, they may leak information to the press. I can't have that."

"What do you suggest?" Simon asked, throwing his hands up in frustration.

"I suggest you announce that you will take a sabbatical for a few months," Leach said. "It is not a punishment, but we need to let things cool down."

"I've never taken a sabbatical," Simon said.

"It might do you good. I know you received your medical degree in Strasbourg which is also Cynthia's home town. Perhaps a trip to your alma mater would be of interest."

Simon laughed bitterly. "Although I did meet my wife there, I hated every second away from London. No medical school here in England would take me."

"Enough of this. Find a place to disappear to for a while. As a friend. Please."

"Well, from school in Strasbourg, I do have friends in Vienna and Budapest," Simon said, shaking his head.

The visit to Strasbourg lasted a week. Cynthia's parents had both passed but she had a plethora of cousins to visit. Simon couldn't leave fast enough.

At that time, Vienna was the medical capital of the world, also noted for its opera, ballet, and symphony. They attended lectures at the medical school during the day and arts performances at night.

Budapest had the reputation of a poor man's Vienna, but Simon was anxious to visit. He had sent a letter to a close medical school friend who had departed Strasbourg for Budapest to practice and teach surgery. The friend, Professor Arvyn Gelfand, invited Simon,

Cynthia and Rachel to his house their first night in town to dine with some of his surgical friends and their wives.

As much of the world's medical literature at the time was written in German, all the guests and the Romains had a working knowledge of medical and conversational German.

At the party, they met Dr. Ignaz Semmelweis, an obstetrician, who was about to publish his life's work, entitled, *The Etiology, Concept, and Prophylaxis of Childbed Fever.*[10]

Rachel approached Semmelweis after the introduction. "My mother died of childbed fever when I was one. I am now a surgical nurse and putrefaction[11] or infection is our biggest fear. I can't see how childbed fever would be any different from the wound infection after any simple procedure which almost always leads to death."

"You're probably correct, but it would need to be proven. The one thing I am sure of," Semmelweis said, "is childbed fever is not from miasma,[12] a foolish notion first expounded by Hippocrates in 400 BC."

"But that's what we've been told," Rachel said.

"I have proved beyond any reasonable doubt that miasma is a fallacy," Semmelweis said with clenched fists, "and that infection has to do with the absence of cleanliness during the procedure. I don't know why that is, but the data speaks for itself."

"I want to hear more," Rachel said as the dinner bell

---

[10] Ignaz Semmelweis: was an early pioneer of antiseptic procedures and was described as the "savior of mothers." His work predates Joseph Lister extolling the virtues of sterility in surgery.

[11] Putrefaction/Infection : Putrefaction is the process of decay or rotting in a body or other organic matter. Infection is from the Latin 'to spoil or stain.' Infection by bacteria or any microorganism hadn't been described yet, so physicians believed wound infection was 'putrefaction.' Bacterial wound infection wouldn't be described until the late 1860s and wouldn't be universally accepted until the late 1880s.

[12] Miasma: 'Bad air' or 'night air' was thought to be the origin of infection.

rang. “Might we talk after dinner?”

“Better yet, I am giving a lecture on this topic at the Budapest University of Medicine tomorrow at 1 p.m.”

“May I attend even if Simon cannot?” Rachel asked. “I believe my aunt and uncle had planned a trip to see the synagogues of Budapest.”

“That doesn’t interest you?” Semmelweis asked.

“Not as much as the topic of your lecture,” Rachel said. “Besides, the synagogues will be there the day after tomorrow as well.”

Semmelweis laughed, saying, “Yes, of course they will. You are quite something. You’ll come to the lecture as my personal guest.”

When Rachel told Simon of her plans, he took her aside and said, “Our host tells me Semmelweis is a gifted obstetrician but some sort of contrarian, disbelieving in basic principles. He was forced to leave Vienna, where he taught, based on his disbelief of miasma.”

“I want to hear what he has to say,” Rachel insisted. “If for no other reason than my mother died of childbed fever.”

The next evening, Rachel returned to the hotel at 5 p.m. to find Simon and Cynthia waiting for her in their conjoined suite.

“The lecture finished hours ago! We worried something happened to you,” Cynthia cried.

“It did. I had an awakening,” Rachel said, taking off her coat. “Some medical students and I stayed afterward to talk to Dr. Semmelweis. He’s made me a believer in his theories.”

“Those are his opinions,” Simon said. “Many, even friends, don’t agree.”

“Everyone can have opinions,” Rachel said sharply. “For me, I think the strudel is better in Budapest than in Vienna. But Dr. Semmelweis has data and facts. I cannot see why people aren’t listening to him.”

"We have two hours until dinner. Why don't you share what you've learned?"

"Fine," Rachel said with a smile, "but after dinner I'm going to a party. The medical students invited me."

"We don't know them," Cynthia said. "Is this a good idea?"

"They're harmless Jewish medical students who work under Dr. Semmelweis and Dr. Gelfand," Rachel said. "I thought one, a Johann Swartzberg, was quite handsome, though he may have thought too much of himself. Anyway, I can take care of myself. I'll write the address of the party if you're worried."

"Okay," Simon said with a shrug, knowing Rachel would do what she wanted to do. "But let's hear what Semmelweis told you."

Rachel, excited, began, "His work started at the General Hospital in Vienna. He was curious why so many women were dying of childbed fever. The hospital had two maternity wards, one run by doctors, all men, and another run by midwives. The death rate from childbed fever in the doctor's ward was fifty percent higher than the rate for the midwives."

"Interesting. What did he think was the cause?" Cynthia asked.

"He watched both wards, looking for differences in practice. Positioning the women in labor differed from one ward to another. A priest walked through the doctor's ward but not the midwives' ward. He changed the positioning, but the death rate remained the same. Likewise when he removed the priest."

"I would swap wards," Simon said.

"He did that next. The doctors, when presented with his findings, thought the bad air, or miasma, coming through the windows on their side of the hospital differed from the wind coming through the midwives' side. So they swapped wards."

"What happened?" Cynthia asked.

"The ward switch made no difference," Rachel said.

"He was befuddled and had no answers."

"Go on," Simon said, leaning closely in excitement.

"When a close friend, a pathologist, died of a finger infection after sustaining a cut while doing an autopsy on a woman with childbed fever, he wondered how the two deaths could be connected. His friend's symptoms, the look of the wound, even the fevers were similar, but in a different location. He concluded that something from the autopsy, perhaps a piece of the corpse too small to see, had gotten onto the scalpel or on his hand and caused the infection. It was not miasma or bad air."

"How could he prove that?" Cynthia asked.

"The corpses smelled of rotting flesh and hand soap did not rid the odor from his hands or clothing. However, chlorine solution did. So he ordered his staff to start scrubbing their hands, fingernails, and instruments with calcium hypochlorite[13] between each patient until no smell could be detected."

"Their hands would turn to leather with all that chlorite, not to mention inhaling it or getting in your eyes," Cynthia said.

"Perhaps," Rachel said, "but both childbed fever and the death rate fell even lower than the midwives' rate, to only one percent."

"Amazing! Did he present his findings?" Simon asked.

"Of course," Rachel said, "and they thought him crazy."

"I might have as well," Simon said.

"No one would listen. He got angry, made a few influential enemies, and was asked to leave his teaching position in Vienna. So he came home and got a position at the General Hospital of Budapest and repeated his studies."

"And?" Simon asked.

"The data was the same. One percent," Rachel said,

---

[13] Calcium hypochlorite is similar to bleach but more powerful. It is used today for water purification in swimming pools. It is a strong irritant to the eyes and lungs.

“The rate of childbed fever was the lowest in Europe. A few listened. Most did not.”

“It sounds very interesting. Infection is the bane of our existence,” Simon said. “What next?”

“He’s publishing a book on his findings and will return to Vienna to present the data,” Rachel said.

“Tis a shame for the good doctor, he is a marked man,” Simon said. “No matter what he presents, they will not believe him.”

“That’s sad, if true,” Rachel said.

“That’s life,” Simon said.

“When we return home,” Rachel said, “I think we should test some of his theories and see how it turns out. Dr. Semmelweis gave me the recipe for the scrubbing solution.”

“Perhaps,” Simon said, “but to prove the point, we’d need hundreds of patients with similar conditions, such as one finds in a maternity ward. We don’t have those kinds of numbers. All the patients have different findings and anatomical locations.”

“You won’t even try?” Rachel said.

“I don’t know,” Simon said. “It will make for more work.”

“Oh, Simon,” Cynthia said, “see how excited Rachel is. I, for one, will try.”

“Alright, alright,” Simon said. “The women in my life are revolting. I have no choice but to surrender.”

After dinner, Rachel changed clothes, removed Andrew’s engagement ring, and left for the medical student party. She returned in less than an hour.

“Home early. What happened?” Cynthia asked.

“Fools, the lot,” Rachel said as she threw her coat on the suite’s sofa. “They didn’t believe I ever lived on a boat. They didn’t believe I could become a doctor or a surgeon if given the chance. None of them would ever marry a woman who even tried. Johann Swartzberg was the worst of all. The other women at the party agreed with him. So I told them what I thought of their closed mentality, and then I left."

"Good for you," Cynthia said.

"The students may say something to Dr. Gelfand about you," Simon said. "I'll make sure he knows your background to set them straight."

"I don't give a toss," Rachel said, as she entered her bedroom. "We'll be gone before that happens. Fools, the lot of them. I can't wait to go back to England. Good night." Even with the door closed, the word "Fools," floated into the room, loud and clear.

Cynthia snickered. "I wonder how she truly feels."

Simon laughed, then whispered to Cynthia, "I think I miss Andrew."

Cynthia's face grew solemn as she nodded agreement and whispered back, "I know she misses him too."

Chapter Twelve
Surgeon – May, 1861 London

Upon their return to England, Simon made it clear to Rachel that she would be unable to perform surgical procedures; he didn't want Sir Archibald Leach breathing down his neck again. Rachel accepted this without comment, spending her first few days back in the hospital obtaining calcium hypochlorite solution bottles and scrub brushes. She placed these throughout their private clinic and outside the operating suites and wards in the Royal London Hospital – much to the annoyance of the other doctors and surgical nurses.

Within forty-eight hours, Leach called Simon to his office.

"What is your game now?" he asked. "The nurses refuse to scrub their hands with chlorite and both doctors and nurses find the odor offensive."

Simon said, "May I explain?"

"By all means," Leach said.

Simon explained the theories of Ignaz Semmelweis in detail while Leach shook his head during the entire dissertation.

Leach asked, "Do you want my opinion?"

"Of course," Simon said.

"You've been hoodwinked. And I'll not force the staff to endure such nonsense. If you want to use Semmelweis's Solution or whatever you call it, then limit it to your own clinic and operating suites. If, and only if, your wife and niece are the only two in the room."

"But, Sir Archibald ..."

"No buts," Leach interrupted. "I have a hospital to run and no one wants this."

Simon started to speak, but Leach held his hand up. "Understood?"

Simon nodded.

"And I don't need to tell you," Leach continued, "that your niece is not a surgeon, she's a nurse. Don't get confused, unless you want a more permanent sabbatical."

Leach then shooed Simon out of his office like a disgruntled diner moving a fly off his supper.

When Simon, affronted, explained to Rachel and Cynthia how his meeting with Leach had gone that afternoon, Rachel shook her head in disgust and said, "I see now how poor Dr. Semmelweis was treated. No wonder he was frustrated."

"It is what it is, I'm afraid," Simon said. "I could seek privileges at another hospital, but we'll run into the same obstacles with hypochlorite and Rachel will still not be able to do more than assist."

"That's too bad," Cynthia said. "She was so excited to do the experiment."

"She's right here and she's bloody irritated," Rachel snapped. "We could be saving lives!"

"Language!" Cynthia said.

"If none of the other surgeons or nurses are willing to try," Simon said, "we'll fail for lack of numbers and lack of control. We won't know what the ward nurses will be doing when we're not around. I see the trial doomed from the onset."

"Let's just us try it anyway, just to see how it goes with us," Rachel pleaded. "I so want to make a difference."

Simon nodded acquiescence.

A week later, as the Romains sat for dinner, Rachel said, "I believe I left Andrew's engagement ring in a cupboard in the nurse's dressing room. I'm going to head back and see if I can find it."

"You don't think it will be there in the morning?" Simon asked.

"Probably, but I won't sleep worrying about losing it," Rachel said.

Cynthia said, "I'll come with you and help look."

Rachel smiled, touched by Cynthia's recognition of the ring's importance to her.

Simon said, "Then if it's all right with you ladies, I'll head over to the club for a game of whist."

"Be careful how much you drink," Cynthia said. "You've cases to do tomorrow morning."

"Yes, Mother," Simon said with more than a trace of sarcasm.

At 8 p.m., Rachel and Cynthia arrived at the surgical nurse's dressing room with kerosene lanterns in hand.

"Mum, you head down this aisle and I'll take the next," Rachel said.

Cynthia found the ring in the third cupboard she inspected. "Got it."

Rachel ran around to find Cynthia and put on the ring immediately. She gave Cynthia a long hug.

"I know you miss him, don't you?" Cynthia said.

"Yes. So much."

As they exited the dressing room, a loud scream emanated from the operating suites down a hallway.

"Help! Help!"

They saw a nurse, Barbara Gubbay, whom Cynthia and Rachel both knew as Sir Archibald Leach's assistant, hurrying down the hallway toward them. Gubbay, from Dorset County, was an experienced senior surgical nurse at the Royal London Hospital who seldom showed emotion. It was disorienting to see her so agitated.

"What's wrong, Barbara?" Cynthia asked as she forced the rushing nurse to stop.

Gubbay, out of breath, said in a rush, "Sir Archibald was in the middle of repairing an incarcerated umbilical hernia. After exposing the hernia, he stepped back from the operating table to sneeze. He tripped over a stool, hit his head on the floor, and raised quite a large flap of scalp. He's not himself and can't continue. I believe he's suffered a concussion."

Understanding at once, Cynthia asked, "Are there

any other surgeons on the ward?"

"I'm going to look but there were none an hour ago! The man is anesthetized and his hernia exposed."

"How can we help?" Rachel asked.

"I need to locate a surgeon. Is Mr. Romain with you or near about?"

"No. He's off to play cards at his club and will have had a significant amount of spirits in him by now," Cynthia responded.

"Please, might you go into the operating suite and see to Dr. Leach whilst I look for another surgeon on the wards?" Gubbay begged.

"Yes, of course we will," Rachel said. "You'll need to return immediately if you find no other surgeons."

Gubbay ran off as Cynthia and Rachel returned to the dressing room, removed their jewelry and rings, dressed into surgical gowns, scrubbed their hands with hypochlorite, then rushed into the operating suite. Sir Archibald was slumped on the floor in the corner with his head bandaged. The anesthetist, Dr. Kenneth Lloyd, had the patient's face under a chloroform mask. Cynthia went to Sir Archibald and Rachel went to the anesthetized patient.

"Cynthia, Rachel, did Mrs. Gubbay find another surgeon?" Dr. Lloyd asked.

"She's looking," Cynthia said.

Cynthia found Sir Archibald seemingly asleep and snoring. Her attempts to awaken him met with grunts, moans and whispered complaints of "Leave me be."

Rachel, standing at the patient's side, was examining the open incision and the incarcerated hernia when Gubbay re-entered the operating suite.

"This is bad," Rachel said. The incarcerated bowel is quite dark and getting no blood flow."

"Worse, there are no surgeons on the ward," Gubbay said breathlessly. "Mr. Alanis lives only a mile from the hospital. I will look for a cab at this hour and go to his home hoping to find him there."

“This man needs the hernia reduced before the bowel becomes necrotic and perforates,” Rachel said. “I know what to do.”

Gubbay grimaced, lowering her voice to a whisper. “We've all heard you were operating on Mr. Romain's cases. Do you think you actually know what to do?”

“Yes,” said Rachel shortly, “and it must be done now.”

“God help us,” Lloyd exclaimed.

“Go ahead then,” Gubbay said, “and pray that I find Mr. Alanis in time. Stop if you believe you're putting the patient's life in jeopardy.”

Gubbay ran from the suite.

Fifty-five minutes later, Mr. Oscar Alanis, an experienced surgeon, raced into the operating room trailed by Barbara Gubbay. They both looked at Sir Archibald, head bandaged, still appearing unconscious in a corner of the room on the floor. They then approached Rachel and Cynthia, who were standing on each side of the anesthetized patient.

“How can I help?” Alanis asked, looking over Cynthia's shoulder as Rachel put in the last suture to close the skin.

“Nothing to do now,” Cynthia said. “The incarcerated bowel has been reduced and the hernia repaired using silk sutures. The incarcerated bowel appeared healthy and pink once the pressure was relieved.”

“Who did the procedure?” Alanis asked.

“I did,” Rachel said.

“Impossible,” Alanis declared, going purple. “You're a nurse, not a surgeon.”

“Don't raise your voice,” Cynthia said. “She's a nurse who happens to know how to reduce the bowel and repair the hernia. We happened to be in the hospital when this happened.”

The anesthetist, Dr. Lloyd, spoke up. “Oscar, I watched and I must say that Miss Romain was more than competent. In fact, she worked quite effortlessly, in my opinion."

"Impossible," Alanis repeated.

"Would you have expected me to keep the man asleep for hours?" Lloyd asked, "whilst Mrs. Gubbay searched the streets for a surgeon, not knowing whether she would find one? The gentleman's abdominal incision was open and the herniated bowel looked as dark and cold as a witch's heart. I've seen a few whilst giving anesthetics."

"No one needs to know who operated," Rachel said.

"I, for one, will not take credit or blame," Alanis said. "If the man dies, I want no responsibility."

"Then Sir Archibald repaired the hernia, closed the incision, and then fell over the stool," Cynthia said. "He won't remember it."

"I'm leaving and was never here," Alanis declared as he turned and exited the suite.

When the patient awoke, Rachel and Cynthia placed him on a gurney and Mrs. Gubbay transported him to the surgical ward. Cynthia and Rachel stayed with Sir Archibald, trying to revive him.

Thirty minutes later, Sir Archibald had regained his senses. "Who repaired the hernia?" he cried. "Did Simon come?"

"No, he was away and no other surgeons nearby," Cynthia said. "Rachel reduced the bowel and repaired the hernia. She used the techniques Simon had taught her. Only after the skin had been closed did Mr. Alanis appear."

"I don't believe it," Sir Archibald repeated as Mrs. Gubbay returned to check on him.

"Then ask Mrs. Gubbay," Rachel said.

Mrs. Gubbay explained the two hours after he had fallen, including Dr. Alanis' arrival and departure.

"Thank you, then," Sir Archibald said, "but this is going to be a problem. Alanis will tell everyone. He was one of the doctors who complained about Miss Romain operating."

"Better to have left the man on the table?" Cynthia asked.

"No. But still a problem that will need to be dealt with. As long as you're here, would you look at my scalp?" Sir Archibald asked.

Rachel and Cynthia agreed, laid Sir Archibald on a table and washed the wound with salt water. Seeing no active bleeding, Rachel used dissolvable gut sutures to close the wound. Once done, they escorted Sir Archibald home in a cab.

When Cynthia and Rachel returned home at midnight, they found a distressed Simon waiting in the parlor and quickly related the entire episode. Looking troubled, he said: "There may be hell to pay. Alanis is not to be trifled with. He covets Sir Archibald's job and would like nothing more than to report this episode to the press."

"What do we do?" Rachel asked.

"Nothing. All we can do is wait for Sir Archibald to invite us to his office. I fear what might become of the three of us."

Overcome with regret, Rachel cried, "I should have never allowed you to teach me surgery!"

"Perhaps," Cynthia said. "But you were marvelous tonight. You took charge of an impossible situation. Like it or not, a surgeon is what you are."

When the three Romains arrived at Sir Archibald's office a week later, they discovered it packed. Sir Archibald sat at his desk, while Mrs. Gubbay, Dr. Lloyd, and Mr. Alanis sat on chairs in a semicircle around the desk. The Romains took the three remaining seats, with Cynthia and Simon on each side of Rachel. Mrs. Gubbay flashed them a quick, sympathetic smile, then quickly looked down at her lap.

"Thank you for coming," Sir Archibald said. "We have a tricky situation to deal with today. One good thing is that I've now talked to all of you who were present at this unfortunate turn of events, and your stories are identical. Another positive is that both the patient and I have survived, our wounds are healing, and the hernia patient knows nothing of what happened."

"I assume the bad things will come next," Simon whispered to Cynthia.

Sir Archibald continued. "The worst thing is that an unlicensed person, Miss Romain, performed surgery at our institution. This could result in our hospital losing its charter and donors. Not the mention the young lady could go to jail. In a court of law and in front of the licensing commission, the particulars are so unusual that this ordeal might be passed over. *Might.* But if word of this gets into the newspapers, the authorities will get involved whether we like it or not."

Sir Archibald waited, scanning the faces of his colleagues. "I don't like uncertainty, so I've settled on a plan that will satisfy everyone to some degree. I've spent most days this past week working out the details. Please, hold your comments until you've heard the plan in its entirety."

Rachel took hold of Simon and Cynthia's hands and squeezed.

"First, everyone in this room must agree this story will never see the light of day. Our lips will and must be sealed. Agreed?"

Everyone nodded. Simon watched Mr. Alanis, who nodded with a subtle smile on his face. Simon instinctively understood that Alanis already knew and agreed with the details of Sir Archibald's plans, or the press would be hawking the story by now.

"Next, my recent accident, perhaps, is a harbinger of things to come for me. I will be sixty-five this July, and I think it is high time for me to retire my position so my wife and I are free to do some traveling. As of tomorrow, Mr. Alanis has agreed to take over my duties as

Chairman of the Department of Surgery. We had hoped to visit our daughter in Charleston, South Carolina, but, as you all may have heard, war has broken out between the Northern and Southern states. How stupid England was to have let the colonies go! This never would have happened under our rule."

Rachel leaned over to Cynthia and whispered, "I don't give a damn about his travel plans or bloody America. I'm madder than hell."

"Shhh ..."

"I won't be...." Rachel started.

Sir Archibald looked at Rachel and Cynthia, which redirected their attention front and center. He then looked to Mr. Alanis. "Oscar, congratulations on your new position. You may leave now, as I have to deal with Miss Romain."

Alanis smiled at the group, then exited the office. Rachel gripped the arms of Cynthia and Simon, expecting the guillotine blade to fall at any moment.

Leach turned his attention to Rachel. "Everyone, let me finish before commenting. Miss Romain, you have broken the law and will no longer be able to assist in any surgical procedures at The Royal London Hospital."

Rachel let go of Cynthia's arm and opened her mouth to voice a complaint but Simon squeezed her other hand and whispered, "Wait."

Leach continued. "Some time ago, you asked me why women could not be doctors or surgeons. I gave you a response that I thought to be true at the time. You've demonstrated that I was in error. I've talked with Dr. Lloyd who told me how expertly you handled a very difficult situation with great poise and skill and, at the same time, saved my reputation. So, thank you for that."

Rachel merely nodded, unsure where Leach was heading.

"Anyway, being knighted and having Queen Victoria as a patient gives me a fair amount of latitude as how to deal with you. I've talked to the board of the new charity hospital, St. James Charity, opening this month in the East End of London. No surgical practitioners, for obvious reasons, practice in the impoverished East End or wish to be on the full time staff of a charity facility. When I told the board of Miss Romain's surgical skills, they said they would work out an arrangement with the City of London so you will be the only surgeon on staff at the hospital. St. James is a charity hospital, so the salary will be only twenty-five pounds per year."

Sir Archibald looked toward Simon and added, "Of course, St. James Charity expects to have London's private surgeons donate time and expertise as needs arise."

Rachel, too stunned to breathe, put both hands to her mouth.

"If any of you don't agree to this plan, speak up now," Sir Archibald said.

No one said a word.

Sir Archibald said, "This meeting will now adjourn and, as we all promised, mum is the word."

Dr. Lloyd and Barbara Gubbay congratulated Rachel on her new position before leaving. Rachel then approached Sir Archibald. "Thank you, Sir Archibald," she said. "This is more than I could have hoped for."

"You saved a patient's life and me from terrible embarrassment at the end of my career," Sir Archibald said. "The board at St. James Charity Hospital will evaluate your work. If you don't pass muster after a trial period, they may need to find another surgeon. As you will be paid almost nothing and it is a charity hospital, I suspect they will not look or evaluate too strenuously."

"She won't disappoint the board or you, Sir Archibald," Simon said.

"I know that now," Sir Archibald said. "Good luck to you all."

Chapter Thirteen
To the South

Following her first successful year at St. James, gaining the admiration of the staff and visiting surgeons who helped further her surgical training, Rachel applied for membership in the Royal College of Surgeons, believing her apprenticeship with Simon, her experience with visiting consultants at St. James, and finally her outstanding record fulfilled her qualifications. However, the College denied her membership on the basis of her not having formally attended a medical school. This despite the fact that no English medical schools accepted Jews or women.

Cynthia continued to look for potential suitors for Rachel. The few Cynthia found never called a second time. From what Cynthia could glean from her friends, Rachel simply intimidated most men. She was a surgeon, spoke her mind, and lacked the refinements in demeanor and language that most men expected. Rachel seemed not to care that none asked to see her again.

Sadly for Rachel and Simon, attempts to institute Ignaz Semmelweis's recommendations at St. James Charity Hospital also failed. Although willing to listen to their arguments, the hospital board, the nurses, and the visiting surgeons refused to participate in any changes. At St. James Charity Hospital Board meetings, other physicians argued that surgical procedures differed from patient to patient. To attain the high numbers of identical cases needed in order to compare data bordered on the impossible.

After one such meeting, Dr. Michael Diamond, a medical physician on the board of St. James, told Rachel in a jest, "What you need is an invasion of England by a foreign power with mass casualties."

Over dinner that night, Rachel told Simon of Dr. Diamond's offhand remark then added, "Do you think we can get the French to invade anytime soon?"

The laughter at the table brought Sharron running into the dining room to find the cause of such glee. When told of Rachel's comment, she joined the laughter.

"There is another way, I suppose," said Cynthia hesitantly, once the laughter had died down. "The papers here tell of horrific battles and casualties in the American Civil War. The numbers of deaths and injuries belie belief."

"Interesting thought," Simon said.

"I'm sorry I brought it up. No way am I going to America," Cynthia said. "Even the short trip across the English Channel leaves me with an ill stomach for days. "I love that Rachel adores the sea, but that's as close as I'll ever get to a body of water bigger than a bathtub."

With that, the room erupted with laughter again.

The next morning, just as Simon and Rachel were about to leave for work, Rachel said, "Mum's comment about the war in America has some merit. Would you think it wise if I tried to go abroad to replicate Dr. Semmelweis's theories?"

Simon, lacing his boots, paused.

"Five obstacles immediately come to mind," Simon said. "First, you'd need to get some kind of United States government approval that you'd be allowed to do the research before even stepping on a ship. Second, it'll be expensive."

"This is my idea. I'd use money from my trust."

"Thirdly, Cynthia won't let you go. Fourthly, even if you could get her to agree, Cynthia wouldn't let you go alone. And lastly, I don't want to go."

"Why would mum block my wishes?"

"She would see too many risks in you entering a battle zone alone."

"Then it's still possible," Rachel said. "I've read about Crimea. There is no strategic value in attacking a hospital. Most of the men will be dead, dying, or unable to fight again, while the doctors and nurses aren't about to mount a charge."

Simon responded, "War is unpredictable and uncivilized. Sanitation may be non-existent. There are too many risks."

"Would you be against me writing to the American Armies, using your name and reputation as a Fellow in the Royal College of Surgeons, asking if they would allow us to aid the injured men whilst doing our research?"

"You'd need to write letters only to the North. I know for a fact the Northern states have blockaded the ports of the Southern states. That's why the prices of cotton goods are so dear. If the Northern states agree, that's the place to go."

"Then I'll write only to the North."

"It doesn't hurt to write," Simon said, then added, "I have little idea how backward American army medicine might be. One can only hope someone over there has read Florence Nightingale's *Notes on Nursing* on the need to improve sanitation in the British Army. Don't for one second get your hopes up that they will accept your proposal."

Rachel wrote a letter to the Department of War in Washington, D.C. and mailed it after Simon had inked his signature.

Ten weeks later, they received a response from the Union Army. Dr. William Hammond, Surgeon General of the United States, and Dr. Jonathon Letterman, Medical Director of the Army of the Potomac, both signed the letter, leaving no doubt about how they viewed Rachel's proposal.

July 1, 1862
Mister Simon Romain
c/o The Royal London Hospital
London, England

Dear Mister Romain,
The United States Army received your

and your niece's request to perform experiments on our troops. We have no time for such nonsense.

In addition, as your experiment gives succor to the enemy, you will not be given permission to enter or provide aid to any of the illegal Confederate states.

Dr. William Hammond, Surgeon General of the United States

Dr. Jonathon Letterman, Medical Director of the Army of the Potomac.

Simon showed the letter to Rachel, who could only shrug at the admittedly predictable response.

"I was so excited to test Semmelweis's theories," Rachel said with a pouty look, "but the gods don't seem to be with me."

"The gods weren't with Semelweiss either," Simon said. "If we can't answer the 'why', then many will dismiss our findings as they did with Semmelweis."

"But even if we don't know why it works, at least we can save lives. No?"

"Yes," Simon said. "Yes, we can. But be prepared to fight to get people to listen. It's happened before, and not just with your friend Semmelweis. Edward Jenner proved beyond doubt that cowpox vaccination prevented smallpox in the 1790s."

"Of course. We've all been vaccinated," Rachel said.

"Jenner proved his theory," Simon said, "but it took decades before widespread cowpox vaccination was accepted. The reason, I believe, was that Jenner couldn't explain why it worked. We still don't know."

"Damn," Rachel said.

"We can't get that word out of your vocabulary, can we?"

"When a better word for an insufferable situation arises, I'll use it," Rachel said. "I won't give up. I will write a letter to the South, blockaded or not."

Rachel confirmed that mail from Europe could not be sent to Richmond, Virginia, the capital of the Confederacy, because of the naval blockade. She approached a merchant, Thomas Knapp, at his huge warehouse near the Thames. Rachel, used to the smell of open sea and the squawking of fat gulls, recoiled at the river's rancid odors of human waste, industrial sewage and the dead animals floating toward the North Sea. It wouldn't be until 1875 that the new London sewer system would be in place.

Rachel had met Knapp at her father's memorial service. Knapp told her he had used her father and the *Sol Quest* to ship and receive goods from the Far East and Africa.

Rachel presented her plan and the dilemma of getting a letter to Richmond, Virginia, to Knapp.

"I know a gun runner, Harold Haas," Knapp said, "a beastly, outrageous, ship captain if ever there was one. He says whatever comes to mind, regardless of the consequences."

"Sounds like a pirate," Rachel said. "Is he trustworthy?"

"He's honest with me and that's all I care about. I'm sure he knew your father. These days, he quite successfully smuggles arms and gunpowder into Wilmington, North Carolina from England and Havana, then returns to England with cotton. He's making money hand over fist. He tells me that his ship is lighter and faster than the Union ships and once inside Wilmington harbor, he's safe. I expect to see him in the next week or so. He usually leaves for the Americas a fortnight after arriving in London."

"Do you think he could transport a letter from me to Richmond, Virginia?" Rachel asked.

"I see no other way," Knapp said. "It's a war, so when, how, or if you get an answer might be a bigger issue. I'd recommend having the response mailed back to Mr. Haas in Wilmington. He'll then bring the letter back to England, or mail it from Jamaica or Havana."

"So complicated," Rachel said.

"A letter is one thing. How you and Mr. Romain would get into the southern states unharmed might present a bigger challenge."

"One step at a time," she said with a smile.

Four months passed and Rachel had abandoned hope of doing her experiment. On arrival home one night, however, Simon said, "A Mr. Knapp dropped off a letter addressed to me, but we know it's for you. It's sitting in the parlor."

Simon followed Rachel into the parlor, where she opened the letter dated three months earlier, and read aloud.

August 12, 1862
Mister Simon Romain
c/o The Royal London Hospital
London, England

Dear Mr. Romain,

We received your request to study the effects of personal sanitation with sodium hypochlorite on surgical patients and will try to accommodate you however possible. We invite you to come to Richmond to work out the details of your research.
Be aware that we offer no equipment, money, or assistants in this endeavor.

Sincerely,
Dr. Samuel Preston Moore
Surgeon General of the Confederate States of America.

"What do you think?" Rachel asked, beaming.

"If it were easy and safe to do, I'd be supportive," Simon said. "Only, how do we get to Richmond if the ports are blockaded? A patient told me the only reasonable and safe option is to sail to Mexico and try to enter the Texas territory, then head east."

"That would take months and months," Rachel complained, throwing herself down on the parlor's sofa. "The war could be over by then. The captain who got the letter into Wilmington is the quickest."

Simon shook his head. "And run the naval blockade? That sounds ridiculously crazy."

Rachel replied, "He seems to be able to do it very successfully."

"We risk being captured, or worse, killed!"

"I am going to go, whether you come with me or not."

Simon sighed; he recognized the stubborn look on her face. "They will not help us in any way," he warned. "We'll need tents, tables, lanterns, bandages, ether or chloroform, and able assistants, not to mention horses and wagons. It'll be very difficult and costly."

"I'm going," she repeated. "I'll buy what I need wherever the gunrunner takes me. I'll notify St. James Charity that I plan to leave as soon as Mr. Knapp's friend, Captain Haas, departs next for the Americas."

Simon sighed.

"Poor Cynthia. She's not going to take this news well."

The next morning at 5 a.m., Rachel arrived at warehouse of Thomas Knapp and Company. Upon entering Knapp's office, she was greeted by the largest, most frightening human being she'd ever encountered. This beast of a man had matted hair, a scar that ran from his left ear to his jaw, and a decided limp. He appeared as tall as a horse and equally as wide. She knew he had to be a sailor by his simple, loose-fitting linen shirt and pants.

"Who's this pretty little thing," the man said too loudly. "Too pretty and too well dressed to be Tommy's whore, but if you be that, I'll buy you off him."

This kind of rudeness got Rachel smiling. She'd heard similar in ports she visited back in her days as Ray. She also knew she couldn't show fear and replied in an instant: "You can shove your thoughts up your bloody arse. I'm here to do business with Mr. Knapp."

The man laughed at Rachel's retort. "Don't get dressed down too oft' by a pretty young thing. Most of 'em run like hell. Might have been fouled up 'bout you. Tommy's not here yet but I reckon he'll be here soon enough. He owes me money. Got my ship almost loaded and the tides are favoring for day after t'morrow or the next."

Rachel realized the letter from the Confederacy had been delivered the day before and she remembered Knapp's description of Harold Haas. This huge mass of flesh fit the description. She gazed upon him anew, with delighted eyes.

"I'm guessing you're Harold Haas?"

"Hmmph. You some kind of spy?"

"You brought a letter from Virginia addressed to my uncle, Simon Romain."

"Well, I'll be damned, you're Jacob's kid," Haas said. "I loved your pa. Good man and treated me fair. Shame 'bout losing him."

"I'm his one and only," Rachel said.

Haas scratched his head.

"I know'd he had a boy too. I know'd that for sure. We crossed paths last in Cape Town, maybe ten, eleven years ago."

"I'm that boy," Rachel said. "Went by Ray then. Fooled everyone."

Haas released a peal of surprised laughter, shaking his head. "Sure fooled me. What business you got with Tommy?"

"My business is with you, actually," Rachel said. "My

uncle and I need to get to the southern states, and quickly."

"You're a bag 'o surprises," Haas said. "Why would anyone wanna go there in the middle of a war?"

"I'm doing medical research. My uncle and I are surgeons and we need to prove a theory. Only a war can provide the kind of proof we need."

Again, Haas roared with laughter. "First she's a sailor, now she's a surgeon! Hard to believe."

"You wouldn't want to wager on it?" Rachel asked. "I could take you over to St. James Charity Hospital in the East End and remove something, like a leg or arm."

Haas belly-laughed at this threat. "Learn something new every day. It'd be an honor then to get you to Wilmington. Least I can do for Jacob."

"Can you wait a week before leaving so we can get some equipment together?" Rachel asked.

"Leave in two days," Haas grumbled, "maybe three. Tides are favorable then and the weather is fair. Otherwise, I'll be stuck here for another two weeks. Won't do that."

"I'll be there," Rachel pledged. "With or without my uncle."

"Since you're Jacob's kid, might you know some answers to rumors floatin' around the docks for last few years?"

"Answers to what?" Rachel asked.

"The scuttlebutt was that a friend o' mine, Jacob's First Mate, Ol' Tom Voz, s'posed to have won the Cowes Week race a few years back with a bunch of army dragoons and maybe a young lass as crew. Nobody seems to know the truth of it all. I remembers Jacob telling me that Ol' Tom was the best there was."

"I know the whole story," Rachel said.

"You'll tell me?" Haas asked.

"Plenty of time on your ship to explain it," Rachel said.

"How do I know you know what happened?" Haas

asked.

Rachel raised her right arm. "Hand to God, Ol' Tom Voz taught me never to lie to a friend." Rachel then spit into the palm of her right hand and extended it to shake.

Haas smiled, spit in his right palm, then shook Rachel's hand which enveloped Rachel's up to her forearm. "Two nights and the next morn and if you're at the St. Katherine's dock, we'll get ya there. Quick stop in Havana, then I'll run you to Wilmington in the Carolinas."

Cynthia, a scowl pasted on her face, accompanied Simon and Rachel to St. Katherine's Dock at 6 a.m. two days later. She had worn that scowl ever since she learned that Rachel and Simon would be leaving on short notice. When the Union army had refused their offer, she'd been hoping that Simon and Rachel wouldn't leave at all.

Cynthia faced Simon as they entered the docks, Rachel having gone off to find Haas' ship. "There are so many ways this could turn into a tragedy," she said. "I would be lost without the two people in the world I love most."

"We'll be fine," Simon said. "I'll watch Rachel like a hawk."

"You can't watch her every second and she has your brother's bad judgment."

"If things turn too perilous, we'll come straight home," Simon said. "That's a promise."

Rachel found Haas' ship, the *Sophia Rose,* and returned to Simon and Cynthia. Simon then went off to find the porter watching their traveling chests and surgical equipment.

Cynthia seized Rachel by the hands and faced her. "You must promise me to take no risks and listen to Simon if he fears danger."

"I promise," Rachel said.

"I trust Simon, "Cynthia said, "and I love you with all my heart. But there's a saying somewhere in the Prophets that we cannot change the spots on a leopard."

Rachel shrugged having no idea what Cynthia meant.

"You have a wild streak which clouds your judgement. Please stay with Simon at all times, no matter what, so he can give you counsel."

"I promise," Rachel said again, but now clearly understanding Cynthia's concern. She hugged Cynthia and said confidently, "I'm not my father. We'll both come home."

The *Sophia Rose* sat in the second berth from the entry, a fine-looking brig at 450 tons and 145 feet long. In many ways she looked like the *Sol Quest,* although the beam was significantly wider. Rachel knew the *Sophia Rose* would be as slow as oozing molasses, even under full sail.

Rachel mumbled to herself as they approached, "This lug is not running a blockade. I wonder what trick Haas has up his sleeve?"

Harold Haas, so big he seemed to block the morning sun, stood under the mainmast as the Romains approached. He shooed four sailors down to retrieve the luggage and crates of equipment. Simon and Rachel said their final, emotional goodbyes to Cynthia, then traipsed up the gangplank.

Haas met them at the top, enveloping Simon in an enormous hug.

"Your brother, Jacob, was a good man," Haas said. "I will get you safely to Wilmington."

"Thank you," Simon said, gasping slightly at the sight of the huge man and his bear hug.

"The tides are in our favor," Haas declared. "Time to shove off."

Thirty minutes later, the *Sophia Rose* was pulled

from her berth using kedges.[14] Once free of the docks, the tide and small triangular sails allowed her to navigate the Thames out to the North Sea.

Rachel soon reappeared on deck barefoot, wearing a brand-new linen sailor's outfit she'd purchased the day before. She joined Haas at the helm.

"I feel free again," she exclaimed. "Happy to help wherever I'm needed."

Haas laughed. "I can see Jacob in you! We'll find things for you to do. You know the days of sailing ships are numbered. Steam will replace us all in the next few decades."

Rachel nodded. "Change comes for us all, good and bad."

"When we're into open sea," Haas said, "you and I will have tales to tell. I doubt we'll finish by the time we make Havana."

Rachel regained her sea legs in no time. She would climb the ratlines to the top of the mainmast twice daily only for the exercise and to the amazement of the entire crew and Simon.

A spate of good weather and favorable winds allowed The *Sophia Rose* to reach Havana in eleven days.

Once docked, Haas, Simon and Rachel watched the crew unload the cargo of munitions for Wilmington to make room for cotton, tobacco and sugar going back to England.

"O'er thar be the ship to Wilmington," Haas said, pointing across the harbor. "She can outrun a diving seahawk."

Rachel spotted a long, low, side-wheel steamer of four hundred tons, with a slight and narrow frame, its length about eight times its beam. Two large side paddles provided all the speed needed to outrun any armed blockade ships. Two short masts stood fore and

---

[14] Kedge: an anchor placed at a distance, then used to reposition a boat by pulling on the line.

aft of the paddles, with a crow's nest for observation on the aft mast. The ship was painted a dull, dark gray color to make it invisible in anything but bright sunlight.

"Looks fast," Rachel said, now knowing the trick up Haas' sleeve.

"Damn fast," Haas replied.

"What's her name?"

"No name. Don't want no one looking for her. Better not to have a name."

Rachel asked. "Why Wilmington? Aren't there closer ports?"

"Wilmington's got a couple o' entrances so I can pick and choose. I buys cotton in Wilmington at two pence a pound," a smiling Haas said, "and sells it in England for two shillings a pound. I get an even better price for the gunpowder I sell in Wilmington. I'm like the pirate, Blackbeard, eh? Three runs to and from Havana to Wilmington and I can fill the *Sophia Rose* and head back to London."

The following morning, Haas, Rachel and Simon boarded the no-name blockade runner and headed north toward Wilmington, keeping far offshore and away from the Union gunships. In the late afternoon of the third day, Haas, abreast of Wilmington, made his run west on a cold, March, moonless night. A man in the crow's nest kept lookout. Every light on the ship had been snuffed out.

The Wilmington harbormaster's men spent each afternoon scouting the inlets to identify where the blockading Union ships were waiting. At exactly four bells in the evening watch, or 10 p.m., the harbormaster's men would signal a light for ten seconds at the safest entrance. Rachel stood with Haas and two other sailors at the helm, looking for a guiding light. In the moonless night, Rachel couldn't make out her hand four inches from her nose. Finally, a light flashed in the distance and then disappeared.

Seeing the light, Haas had the course and went

ahead at flank speed. Suddenly, a shout from the crow's nest put everyone on guard: "I see muzzle flashes broad on the port quarter coming this a' way. Reckon a couple o' thousand yards."

"Oh no, will they catch us?" Rachel asked, as two cannon balls splashed somewhere close enough to be heard but not seen.

"Nah," Haas said. "Those be long shots. Probably a mile away or more. They know we'll be long gone 'afore they get here. They're firing on an empty sea so they can say they tried."

"Still scary," Rachel said.

"Fact is," Haas said, "the Union boats be getting faster and smarter. Lots of runners these days try to beach their boats on the nearest piece o' land when they knows they be caught. If stopped out at sea, they lose everything, boat and cargo. If they beach their boat, they figure the boat's done for but can salvage the cargo on the beach. I'm too smart to let either happen to me."

Haas docked in Wilmington harbor two hours later.

Before leaving the ship, Haas pulled Rachel and Simon aside. "You two will need to be prepared to see some awful things here, especially in the countryside. They treat their black slaves like animals, whipping 'em sometimes for no reason at all. As much as you'd want to, don't say nuttin'. It's the way it is."

The Romains said their farewells to Haas and the crew, and it wasn't long before Rachel and Simon were asleep in rooms at Stemmerman's Inn on Front Street. They awoke with the sunrise, had breakfast and, with help, loaded their crates, luggage and themselves onto carriages and wagons arranged by the hotel. At the rail station, they booked tickets on the W&W Railroad to Richmond, Virginia.

As Rachel and Simon rolled north through lush North Carolina farmland, they gazed with wide, horrified eyes at the sight of slaves toiling in the fields as slave masters, wielding a whip, sat atop a horse watching.

"Disgusting," Rachel mumbled in Simon's ear.

"Yes."

Rachel, with tears in her eyes, turned from the window and buried her head in a nursing manual to compile a list of the commodities they'd need.

Chapter Fourteen
Flora and Bessy
March, 1863 – Richmond, Virginia

The morning after arrival in Richmond, Simon and Rachel walked nine short blocks from the Linden Row Inn on Haroldian Street to look for Samuel Moore, Surgeon General of the Confederate States of America.

Simon and Rachel entered the Thomas Jefferson conceived magnificent, columned building which served as the capitol building for the Commonwealth of Virginia and the Confederate States of America. Once inside, sentries escorted them to the office of Dr. Moore.

"We take no sides in this war," Simon said. "We're interested only in decreasing the rate of infection after battle trauma."

"Fine and dandy," Moore said, looking only at Simon. "When can you start?"

"We've brought our personal surgical equipment and sodium hypochlorite with us," Rachel said, unused to being ignored. "But we are hoping to purchase whatever else we need here."

Moore looked irritated at the interruption.

"Your nurse don't know her manners. This some newfangled British thing?"

"Miss Romain is my niece, sir," Simon said quickly. "She's also the head surgeon at St. James Charity in London. We'll be doing the research together."

"Hard to believe. She knows this is a war?" Moore asked Simon.

"Damn straight I know it's a war," Rachel said defiantly.

Moore shook his head. "Doubt the men are going to cotton to a woman in their ranks. Womenfolk belong at home with the young ones."

"I don't think so," Rachel said, "A soldier with a shattered leg can't afford to be choosy.".

Before Moore could respond, Simon jumped in.

"If our research doesn't bring a lowered infection rate and fewer deaths, you are free to stop the study," he said.

"Can't argue with that," Moore said, nodding in agreement. "I'll tell you what we've got: wagons, tents, surgical tables, stretchers, and linens. Bandages and lanterns are hard to find, but British pounds speak loudly to merchants. Y'all are going to need two horses for each wagon and two more with saddles to ride."

"Do you have ether or chloroform?" Rachel asked.

"Plenty of both for now. We didn't think the war would last more than six months. Y'all will need some nurses. We've none of those and can't spare any troops other than a couple of sentries."

"Where will we be sent," Rachel asked, "and when must we be there?"

"Tell ya what," Moore said, "some around here think you're spies for the Yankees. I don't – yet. How about I don't tell you when and where until you're ready to head out. Not much going on in winter except some skirmishes here and there. General Lee hasn't been whooped yet, so let's say something's coming. I'll give you a month to get what you need. I'll see you mid-April or so."

"Thank you, General," Simon said. "I'll let you know when we're fully equipped."

"Sounds good to me," Moore said. "First, I need to swear you in as members of the Confederate Medical Corps."

"Is that necessary?" Rachel asked. "We're not taking sides."

"Only necessary if you want to stay and do your research," Moore said crankily. "You can return to England right now if you don't."

Simon and Rachel nodded yes. Moore brought out a Bible and had them take an oath to the Confederacy.

Before departing, Moore pulled Simon aside and

said, “May want to have your niece mind her manners a bit. Say less and listen more.”

Anxious to leave, Simon said only, “Thank you.”

After they exited the building, Simon pulled Rachel aside. “We’re in a foreign country. His actions toward you were uncalled for but we’re guests here and if we have any chance of completing our study, you’ve got to settle down.”

“But, he’s...,” Rachel started.

“Yes,’ Simon replied, “he’s a horse’s ‘arse’ in your terms.”

Rachel could only laugh then added, “I could no more take an oath to support their cause than I could for Sodom and Gomorrah.”

“Amen,” said Simon.

After opening a bank account at the Exchange Bank of Richmond on Main Street, Rachel and Simon ate a late lunch at a tavern near the capital. Then they perused the merchants and stables needed to stock their mobile hospital.

“Seems most everything we’ll need is still in fair supply,” Simon said.

“I thought getting horses would be a problem,” Rachel said, “but there’s more than we’ll ever need, secured after battles. I’ve no idea where we’d look for nurses or aides.”

“It’s the back breaking work of cleaning, restocking, and moving injured men we need help with,” Simon said. “We can’t be doing that.”

Rachel nodded agreement. “I’m afraid we’ll need to try to find unskilled men and women and train them on the job. This isn’t London where we can stand on a street corner in the East End and hire ten people in a moment.”

For the next three days, Simon and Rachel scoured Richmond, looking to hire anyone to fill the roles of nurses and aides. The few men or women who needed jobs ran from the interviews when they learned of the work needed, regardless of the pay offered.

On the fourth day of searching, Rachel sat alone in the hotel's restaurant as she finished her lunch. Two well-dressed gentleman in their late fifties, one tall and the other stocky with large protruding ears, entered and took a table near her. Both tipped their hats before sitting and Rachel nodded back. From that point on, neither gave her a glance as they seemed to have problems of their own. Rachel, curious, listened to their conversation.

"You can't be serious about moving north to Cincinnati," the tall man said. "I don't care if your daughter and grandchildren are there. It's a life you aren't fit for."

"Got no other life," the stocky man complained. "My son died at First Manassas under Joe Johnston and my poor Sarah died three months later. There's no one to pass the plantation onto. I don't want to be alone here. I have nowhere to sell my tobacco with the blockade. I've sold or auctioned all but two of my seventy-five slaves to the surrounding plantations at half what they're worth for useless Confederate dollars just to pay off debt."

"Will you find a buyer for your plantation?" the tall man asked.

"Probably not. I'll leave it 'til this damn war's over then come back and see if it has value. Without slaves to do the work, it's only a pile o' dirt."

"How about the house slaves? They might be worth something," the tall man asked.

"The only two remaining are Sarah's upstairs maid, Flora, and her mother, Bessy, the cook. Sarah swore to Bessy before she died that they wouldn't be separated. Bessy said she'd kill herself if we sold Flora off to someone else."

"Who cares what she says," the tall man said. "The next owner will whip her until she changes her mind."

"She's strong willed," the stocky man said. "We sold

her two boys before the war and she took it hard."

"So what'll you do?"

"Take your advice and forget what Sarah promised 'em," the stocky man spat. "I can't take 'em north to Cincinnati, so I'll head over to Brooke and Hubbard's and sell 'em off at the next auction."

"They healthy?"

"Strong as mules, both of 'em. Flora's about seventeen and her ma's maybe thirty-two or three. Both too damn smart for their own good if you ask me."

"Should fetch a few dollars."

The stocky man leaned over and said, "Except Sarah taught both to read and write. No one knows."

"The tall man shook his head. "No one wants to buy an uppity slave who can read."

"I'll kill both of 'em if they let that be known," the stocky man said as the waitress came to take their order.

Rachel paid her bill, exited, then entered the store down the street and asked where she could find Brooke and Hubbard's Auction House. As she walked toward it, she discovered notices pasted to the sides of the buildings announcing the next slave auction would take place in three days.

At the auction house, Mr. Brooke invited Rachel to see the slaves for sale. He mentioned having seen her and Simon about town.

"Y'all not from these parts. Where y'all from?" Brooke asked.

"London."

"That's a fer piece from here," Brooke said.

"My uncle and I are doctors and looking for a pair to help in the house," Rachel said.

"Most of these be field hands," Brooke said.

"On the day of the auction, you'll tell me if such a pair exists?" Rachel asked.

"We've thirty-four blackies for sale as of now. Might be a few more coming in the next day or two. Some families, husband and wife only. Kids and parents are sold separate," Brooke said as he ushered Rachel into a barnlike structure to find all the adult slaves wearing ankle shackles on short chains fixed to the inner wall of the barn.

Rachel blinked hard and took a shallow breath of the acrid smell of human waste, sweat and rotten straw. Only her years as a nurse and surgeon prevented her from vomiting. Haas had forewarned Rachel about the treatment of slaves, but seeing it so close was more that she could tolerate.

Despite the cool spring weather, none of the men and only half the women were fully clothed. All the children under the age of five ran naked and free among those chained. Three-quarters of the men and a few women had scars on their backs from whippings.

As they walked around the barn, coming close to the slaves, Brooke would point his cane at each. The men opened their mouths to show teeth and flexed muscles. The women bowed their heads.

"Feel free to examine or talk to any of these here blackies," Brooke said. "I expect buyers from Virginia, the Carolinas, Georgia, Florida, Alabama and Louisiana. Most of them be speculators who'll take 'em back to their own state and sell 'em for a profit."

"I've seen enough, Mr. Brooke," Rachel said. "Thank you. I'll be back for the auction."

"To buy, you'll need some kind of security guarantee," Brooke said, hitching up his trousers and giving her a smarmy grin. "Can't have you leavin' less you pay up front."

"The Exchange Bank on Front Street holds our money in British Sterling," Rachel said.

"I'd give a discount for British Sterling," Brooke said. "You'll need to put a third down at the sale. You can pay in two installments."

"I'll pay the total in cash at the sale," Rachel said, eager to be free of this odious man.

"My oh my. I need more customers like y'all. Y'all bring a note from the bank, hear. Mr. Anderson or Mr. Joelston." Brooke said. "That'd be enough."

"We met with Mr. Joelston today. That shouldn't be a problem."

When Rachel exited, she needed to sit on a bench to gather her thoughts. She said to herself, 'I wonder how Mr. Brooke would do chained to a wall. I'd like to see that.'

"Are you kidding me," Simon cried, horrified. "We're not buying slaves!"

"Wait until you hear me out. After the auction house," Rachel said, 'I went to an attorney. A Mr. Marvin Siskan. He seemcd quite smart."

"To do what?"

"To determine how one grants slaves their freedom," Rachel said. "It can be done."

Simon's head was in his hands. "President Lincoln already freed the slaves on the first of January. How can you free someone who is already free?"

"I know. I read the papers in London as well. The slaves are free only if the North wins the war," Rachel said. "The Confederate States don't and won't honor anything proclaimed by the North. As we speak, these poor people have no freedom. Siskan told me that even if a slave has valid papers, nobody around here honors them."

"So, what do you wish to do?" Simon asked.

"Give them manumission documents immediately, that's what they're called," Rachel said. "After the war, no matter who wins, technically the slave is free. That's all we can do. If we own them now, we can protect them whilst in the South."

"What'll it cost? This is a huge gamble, I believe," Simon said.

"It could be, and I want to buy both of them," Rachel said. "It looks like we'll find no other help."

"They may not be teachable," Simon said. "Most Londoners can't do what our nurses and aides do. An uneducated slave has no chance."

"I happen to know they can read and write, but no bidder will know that. Apparently teaching them is illegal. I'll promise to keep them together as long as they help us."

"In other words, they're still slaves," Simon said. "Our slaves."

"Please," Rachel said. "We need the help. If they're no use to us, we'll free them however we can. There's another problem, however. I've told the auctioneer, Mr. Brooke, that we're looking for a pair of house help, and he knows we've got the funds to pay in full. According to Siskan, Brooke hires shills in the crowd to keep bidding alive, so the price goes up and up. Brooke then pays the shill off afterward."

"So we're about to go bankrupt over this harebrained scheme to boot?"

"The lawyer, you and I will observe who is bidding against us," Rachel said calmly. "I gave the lawyer twenty British pounds to come to the auction and signal if he thinks a shill is working with Brooke. He'll remove his hat and wipe his brow if he believes the price is too high."

"We have no idea the worth of a slave," Simon said.

"Mr. Siskan filled me in. As a rule, house slaves are worth far less than a strong field hand. Anything more than six hundred dollars for the cook and four hundred for the maid would be exceptional in today's market. Together, that comes to a thousand dollars or five hundred pounds sterling. If I think we're being taken advantage of, I'll let them win. If correct, I'll buy them after the auction for a fraction of the selling price. We'll wait around and the auctioneer will provide some excuse as to why the other buyer wasn't qualified. Anyway, that's what the lawyer told me."

"What if we end up with no one?"

"We keep looking for help. We can always go back to London," Rachel said, "tails between our legs, and say we tried."

Over the next two days, Simon and Rachel purchased four horses, feed, and two saddles from an elderly stable owner named Kim Margoli. From a variety of Richmond merchants, they bought bandages, cooking utensils, personal bedding and vats in which to make the sodium hypochlorite solution. Surgeon General Moore provided wagons, tents, surgical tables, stretchers, and linens.

While Rachel had been riding horses since coming to London, Simon hadn't been on a horse since age eleven. Mr. Margoli gave him riding lessons and then gave both of them cursory lessons on hitching and driving the wagons.

"Y'all have a lot to learn about caring for those there horses and driving the wagon," Margoli said. "Best hope for y'all is the army lends a hand getting y'all from one place to 'nother."

Rachel and Simon said at the same time, "Amen!"

Rachel and Simon went early to the auction site, an elevated platform in front of the Brooke and Hubbard Auction House. Rachel found Mr. Brooke near the auction platform in a jolly mood.

"Mr. Brooke. We met the other day," Rachel said.

"Yes, of course. Y'all looking for house help. What do y'all know but the very next day, exactly what y'all's looking for showed up. A cook and her daughter, a house maid."

"That's wonderful," Rachel said. "When might they be auctioned?"

"They'll bring top dollar," Brooke said, "so I'll have them on the block early while everyone still has money. Bunch of other parties interested in the same."

Rachel returned to Simon, pointing out the attorney, Mr. Siskan, who stood on the other side of the crowd.

"Brooke told me the couple I'm interested in are going to be sold early," Rachel said. "He let me know the bidding will be brisk. I'm already smelling a rat."

As expected, Brooke had Flora and Bessy as the second slaves to be auctioned. Both women were tall, perhaps five foot seven. Bessy, the mother, was dark-skinned while Flora was biracial with large, protruding ears. Rachel could only shake her head, remembering the stocky man in the café with large ears.

As the bidding started, both slaves stood shoulder to shoulder with an arm around the other's waist. They didn't want to be separated.

Brooke spent five minutes extolling the virtues of Flora and Bessy, to be sold as a pair. If the buyer didn't want both, Brooke would auction off the unwanted one.

"Who'll start the bidding at five hundred dollars for the both?" Brooke yelled.

Rachel raised her hand. Immediately, three other hands went up, raising the price to five-fifty, six, then seven hundred. Rachel bid seven fifty. For a moment, no other bids were received. Then, a man at the far back, dressed poorly with mismatched shoes, jumped in at nine hundred. Rachel raised to nine-fifty.

"Does the man at the back have another bid for a thousand?" Brooke said.

The man nodded.

"A thousand it is," Brooke said.

"A thousand-fifty," Rachel said.

"I hope you know what you're doing," Simon whispered.

"Who'll bid eleven hundred," Brooke said.

The man in the back said, "Twelve hundred."

"Something's fishy," Rachel mumbled.

Simon grabbed Rachel's arm and whispered, "Don't look around. Mr. Siskan removed his hat and wiped his brow."

Brooke looked to Rachel. "Twelve fifty is a fair bid for such a fine pair."

Rachel smiled and shook her head. "Let the gentleman have them. We'll not bid again."

Brooke had no option other than yell, "Sold."

With that, Rachel took Simon's arm and walked away. They took a bench across the street where they could still watch the auction which lasted another hour.

Minutes after the auction ended, Brooke approached Rachel and Simon, just as Siskan predicted.

"I think y'all are in luck," Brooke said. "That man who outbid you doesn't have a letter of guarantee from a bank. Those two blackies can be y'all's for twelve hundred dollars."

"Wonderful," Rachel said. "Our last bid was seven-fifty when that scruffy man started bidding it up. I've been to enough auctions to know a shill when I see one. I'll buy them for seven-fifty."

Brooke turned purple. "Y'all stealing those two," he hissed. "They be worth more than seven-fifty."

"Plenty of people were here today," Rachel said without a hint of emotion. "I'll tell anyone who'll listen about this fraud. You'll sell me those two for seven-fifty or else."

Twenty minutes later, Rachel and Simon exited Brooke and Hubbard Auctioneers with two slaves, Bessy and Flora, and their papers of ownership.

Around the corner, Bessy spoke first to Simon. "You our new massa?

"No, my niece, Rachel, will be your new master," Simon said, coughing uncomfortable.

Flora turned to Rachel, urgency in her voice. "Y'all gonna sell us some other place? We wants to stay together."

"We've lots to talk about," Rachel said. "You must be hungry. We'll get some food for you and find a place to sit and talk."

"Y'all talk real funny-like," Bessy said. "Y'all's not

from these here parts."

"My uncle and I are from England. London to be exact. Across the ocean," Rachel said.

"Never heared of that place," Flora said.

Rachel entered a bakery and purchased a loaf of cornbread. Simon then led everyone around the corner on the side of the bakery where he found benches for all to sit. Rachel broke the cornbread loaf in half and offered a half to each woman. The cornbread disappeared in a minute.

"So, y'all from fer away," Bessy said. "I needs to know whatcha gonna do with us."

"First, my name is Rachel Romain and my uncle is Simon Romain. We are doctors and we are here to do surgery on men injured in the war."

Flora and Bessy, confused, looked at each other and shrugged.

"We don't believe in slavery," Rachel continued. "We will go to a lawyer tomorrow and get manumission papers for both of you. That means you'll be free."

Bessy and Flora looked at each other, eyes wide open and more confused than ever.

"If you were in the North, you could go anywhere you want," Simon offered.

"We's got kin in Chicago town," Bessy said. "Dat wheres we go."

"But you're in the South and there's no way to get to the North safely with the war going on," Rachel said. "If you try, the first Southerner that sees you will take you as a slave."

"We knows that," Flora said. "We tried once and the patrol found us four mile from home. Our massa whoop us good." Flora stood, picked up her blouse and showed the scars on her back.

"I'm sorry," Rachel said. "My uncle and I will never whip you or anyone. That's a promise."

Simon nodded agreement. "Never."

"I's confused," Bessy said. "You gots no home or

farm. Why you buys us?"

"We need help with the care of men injured in the war," Simon said. "Cleaning, changing bedding, and cooking, I think. Maybe more."

"Cooking, I can do," Bessy said. "Dats 'bout it."

"I don't do no cooking," Flora said.

"We'll all learn to do everything," Rachel said. "If you want to leave, we won't stop you. However, if you stay and work with us, we will pay you a fair wage of five dollars every week and when the war is over, we promise you safe passage north to Chicago or wherever you want to go."

There was silence.

"I never seen no five dollar in my life," Bessy said, eyes and mouth open.

"Where we gon' stay?" Flora cut in. "Y'all ain't got no house."

"Our hotel has rooms in the basement for you," Simon said. "We'll try to rent a house tomorrow until we head off."

"Head off whereabouts?" Bessy asked.

"Wherever the men are fighting," Rachel said.

"Oh. My oh my. Lord help us," Bessy said.

The next day, Simon secured a month's lease on a six-bedroom house northeast of Monroe Park. The owner, a Confederate officer in Tennessee under General Braxton Bragg, was away in the war and his wife and children had moved to be with her mother in Lynchburg, Virginia. The house came with a caretaker named Theo, an elderly freed slave. The house had a stable big enough for the horses and wagons.

While Simon secured the lease, Rachel went shopping for clothes for Bessy and Flora. Finding no merchant who would allow Bessy and Flora into their store, Rachel found a seamstress to make dresses with white aprons that would serve as nurses uniforms. She also purchased sewing needles, rolls of linen and cotton for Bessy and Flora to make everyday clothing and undergarments. Simon purchased notebooks in which to keep data.

Bessy would cook meals of mutton, pork, and beef dishes, chowders, custards and even bass from the James River. Cornbread appeared at every meal. Despite Bessy's protestations, Rachel helped her cook and helped Flora clean up after the meals.

Bessy and Flora sat with Rachel after the first week's meal.

"I heared the soldiers be eating hardtack and salted pork," Bessy said. "Best I be makin' some o' that for y'all, sos y'all get used to it."

"What's hardtack?" Rachel asked.

"A cracker hard as brick," Flora said. "Good fer knockin' out a loose tooth."

"Sounds good," Rachel said, smiling. "Now there's something else we need your and Flora's help with. When we get busy, Simon and I won't often have time to make notes on the men we treat. We expect you and Flora will be able to keep notes for us."

"Slaves can't read or write, no way no how," Bessy said, shaking her head. "That be agin' the law. People round here sees us readin' or writin', they whip us good. I heared the white folk who teached them their letters could be whipped, pay money, and even do jail time."

"Are you saying," Rachel asked, "that you and Flora don't read and write?"

"I can't says that we do," Bessy said.

"Do you know why we bought you and Flora?" Rachel asked.

"No, Miss Rachel. Didn't make no sense to me or Flora and still don't," Bessy said. "But I thinks y'all gonna tell me now."

Rachel laughed then related how she overheard the conversation in the restaurant of her owner and a friend. "The man told his friend he'd kill you and Flora if anyone found out you both can read and write. Then he wouldn't be able to sell you."

Bessy looked like she'd seen a ghost. "Y'all won't be telling no one, will y'all?"

"No one is going to hurt you or whip you. That I promise," Rachel said. "They'd have to shoot me first."

"White folk can be that mean. They might shoot us and y'all too and not think nothing 'bout it."

"Then you and Flora will have to find a safe place if there are men around. All we need is a name, date, and whether it's a leg or arm. Nothing else. It can be written on a scrap of paper and put in your pocket. We can enter it in a log book at night when we're alone."

Flora looked at her mother and shrugged.

For the next five days, Simon and Rachel practiced mock surgeries while instructing Bessy and Flora as assistants. Rachel tore sheets of a paper into little pieces just big enough for Bessy and Flora to write name, date and procedure when alone. Simon and Rachel created mock charts for each individual listing: name, date of procedure, procedure performed, daily progress, outcomes.

Unsure of how much help with the wagons and horses they could expect, Mr. Margoli and Theo, the caretaker, helped them learn the necessary stable chores.

Chapter Fifteen
Solomon – April 10, 1863

Every few days, Simon would ride to the capital building to meet with Surgeon General Samuel Moore and discuss the status of the war.

"It's good you came by today," Moore said. "We've just learned the Union Army under General Joe Hooker plans to head south from above the Rappahannock River in the next few weeks to confront General Lee. Lee's army has been west of Fredericksburg this winter. You'll need to leave tomorrow or the next day."

"Where should we go?" Simon asked.

"Head to Fredericksburg to meet with Colonel Lafayette Guild[15]," Moore said. "Guild is the medical director of Lee's army. He knows you and your niece are coming and that's about it. I have to be honest; Guild isn't thrilled about you helping out. He thinks you might be more hindrance than help and your niece's presence a fool's mission."

"We won't hinder, that I promise. We'll leave for Fredericksburg as soon as we can load the wagons," Simon said.

"You'll approve of Guild's methods, I think. He's started quarantining soldiers with infectious diseases to some benefit already."

"Good. We think alike then," Simon said.

---

[15] Dr. Lafayette Guild: He graduated from medical school in Philadelphia, then worked in the U.S. Army until the Southern States seceded. He had studied yellow fever extensively while directing health care in New York City on Governor's Island. When isolation of men afflicted with yellow fever did nothing to prevent the spread of disease, he concluded, correctly, that the disease was not contagious like other illnesses. It would not be until the 1890s when Walter Reed proved that mosquitoes were the responsible vector.

Two days later, with packed wagons, Simon, Rachel, Bessy and Flora headed north to Fredericksburg, sixty miles away. Confederate soldiers marching to Fredericksburg lined the road and offered to help drive the wagons. At night, the same soldiers helped Simon pitch tents, unhitch the wagons and feed the horses. In turn, Bessy cooked mutton, pork, and cornbread for the soldiers who helped them.

The trip took two nights and three days before reaching the Army of North Virginia's bivouac west of Fredericksburg and east of Chancellorsville. The trip helped Simon get used to riding a horse for long distances, although Rachel laughed when Simon couldn't sit comfortably on a stool near the firepit for the first night of their relocation.

On the last night before reaching Fredericksburg, a Confederate Major took a liking to Rachel after learning she wasn't actually married. While he spoke to her pleasantly, she later overheard him berating Bessy for overcooking the mutton.

That evening, Bessy waited until Rachel was alone. "I's getting to know y'all, Miss Rachel. Y'all don't want nothing to do with no Southern gentlemen. Theys been raised to hate. Theys hate anyone 'neath 'em. Not just us slaves but po' people too."

"You didn't need to tell me," Rachel said. "I heard the way he talked to you. If we'd been in England, I'd have given him a piece of my mind. Seeing that we need his kind whilst doing our work, I kept my mouth shut."

"You sure is funny," Bessy said. "So you knows, Southern women lets the men do the talking, but they be just as mean."

Upon reaching the outskirts of Fredericksburg, Simon and Rachel rode around for an hour looking for Colonel Lafayette Guild, the medical director of the Army of North Virginia. They found him supervising the conversion of an evacuated large farmhouse into a general hospital.

"Dr. Guild," Simon said, "we're the doctors from England, here to conduct research on war injuries. I'm Mr. Simon Romain and this is my niece, Dr. Rachel Romain. Dr. Moore in Richmond sends his regards."

Lafayette Guild, M.D., in the full uniform of a Colonel in the Confederate Army, looked every bit a man of papers. Tall, handsome, dark-haired, with a well-trimmed beard, Guild exuded confidence.

"Pleasure to meet a member of the Royal College of Surgeons," Guild said to Simon as he shook hands. He tipped his hat to Rachel and added, "Ma'am."

"My niece is an equally qualified surgeon," Simon added.

"But not in the College," Guild noted.

"The College won't allow women," Rachel said. "It has nothing to do with my qualifications or ability." Her jaw tightened. She already didn't like Lafayette Guild.

"Perhaps," Guild said. "We'll see."

The last comment didn't soften Rachel a bit. "Where might we set up our hospital?" she asked.

"We're converting vacant churches and large farmhouses into hospitals. This farmhouse is the fourth and last one we'll convert. As it's the smallest, I'll assign it to you," Guild said. "Field hospitals will be in tents closer to the fighting. Once men are stabilized in the field hospitals, they'll be moved to the general hospitals by ambulance for treatment. Each regiment of three hundred men has two ambulances, carrying four men each, for such transfers."

"Sounds like you've done this before," Simon said.

"Unfortunately, yes," Guild said, bowing his head. "Last September at Antietam, Lee fought McClellan to a draw despite McClellan having twice as many troops. We had over ten thousand casualties in a single day. Our surgeons were overwhelmed."

"Hopefully, our presence will make a difference," Simon said.

Guild shook his head. "I believe that's why Moore allowed you to come when I said no. He felt we needed the help."

"Did anything change after that battle?" Rachel asked.

"We were better prepared for Fredericksburg last December," Guild said, "when Lee destroyed Burnside. Still, we had six thousand casualties in four days. Moore believes the presence of another surgeon will help if the casualty numbers increase."

"Two surgeons," Rachel said.

Guild responded, "So you said. I've read your hypothesis regarding cleansing and isolation to prevent infection after amputation. I've not read or even heard of Dr. Semmelweis. My humble opinion is that you're wasting your time."

"Time will tell," Rachel said. "We plan to keep accurate data to prove or disprove our point."

Guild shrugged indifference with closed eyes and a subtle head shake. "Whatever. When injured men arrive in unimaginable numbers, keeping data becomes close to impossible. At times, we're lucky if we get even a name."

"We understand," Simon said. "We will endeavor to keep it simple. We will accept all injuries as they arrive but we're interested documenting injuries requiring amputations of the arm or leg within forty-eight hours of injury only and nothing else."[16]

Guild shook his head. "You've not been in a war situation yet. You have no idea the chaos that surrounds us. Trust me you won't get a second of sleep for days at a time."

"I understand. In Crimea, the British army reported a twenty-five percent mortality for amputations," Simon said.

"That would be my guess here as well," Guild said.

---

[16] Sixty-thousand amputations were performed during the Civil War, North and South, far and away the most common procedure done.

"If we can show only a five percent mortality," Rachel said. "That would be highly significant."

"You won't," Guild said. "Trust me. Anyway, the surgical teams will meet tonight. You'll be busy setting up here and you don't know where the other general hospitals are located. I'll send messages to the other head surgeons that we'll meet here at sixteen hundred."

Simon and Rachel nodded agreement.

Guild said, "I must be going." He shook Simon's hand. Rachel extended her hand but Guild only nodded, said, "Miss," then turned and departed.

After Guild was out of earshot, Rachel muffled a scream. "My God, what a son of a bitch."

Simon nodded.

"Let's start unpacking," he said with a sigh. "It seems that everyone is going to call me Doctor and you Miss or Ma'am. Don't fight it. It's their land and customs."

Using tables provided by the Confederate quartermaster in Richmond, Simon and Rachel transformed the house's ground-floor rooms into operating theaters. Each room had a sodium hypochlorite station for scrubbing hands and instruments. The cellar would provide storage. The upstairs, accessible only via a narrow stairway, had four small bedrooms. Three would be for Simon, Rachel, Flora and Bessy to use as sleeping quarters. The fourth allowing Flora and Bessy privacy to keep the log books.

"Y'all sure 'bout this," Bessy complained. "We's ne'er sleep nowheres near white folk."

"Where did you sleep?" Rachel asked.

"Small cabin out back the house 'bout as close as we come," Flora said. "That's only times we could talk to one 'nother. Says what we want without gittin' whooped."

"We need to be close to one another," Rachel said. "If there's an emergency, I don't have time to run out to a tent."

"I dunno," Bessy said.

"I do," Rachel said. "Besides, no one is whipping anyone here. We all stay together to protect one another."

"You not like any white woman we's ever knowed of," Flora said. "We give it a try."

"The other head surgeons are coming before dinner for a meeting. Best you make yourselves scarce," Rachel said. "I'll fill you in later."

Bessy and Flora nodded agreement.

At 4 p.m., Colonel Lafayette Guild arrived along with two other surgeons, Colonel John Heath and Captain Jean LeClerc 'Clerk' Jordan.

Heath, forty-seven, overweight, bearded and unhappily clad in an ill-fitting uniform, had been a family doctor in Mobile, Alabama. He joined the army in April,1861, the day he heard South Carolina had shelled Fort Sumter in Charleston Harbor. The Confederacy needed surgeons and Heath watched and learned from Guild and the other surgeons.

Clerk, tall, thin, and clean-shaven, was handsomely dressed. He had graduated medical school in Atlanta in 1862 at the age of thirty-two, after working as a pharmacist in his father's apothecary. Like Heath, Clerk learned to be a surgeon from watching Guild and others. All three had at least six assistant surgeons working under them and ten assistants helping the surgeons with major cases or else doing simple procedures by themselves.

"Dr. Romain, Miss Romain," Guild said, "These are the two other head surgeons, John Heath and Clerk Jordan."

As Guild had done, both Heath and Jordan shook hands with Simon but merely nodded at Rachel, calling her 'Miss.' Rachel began to wonder if shaking a woman's hand was a no-no in the South. They all took seats around a dining table destined to be an operating room table. Guild laid out a map of the region with circles pinpointing the general hospitals.

"General Hooker and the Yankees left Washington yesterday," Guild said. "Only a matter of time before they cross the Rappahannock somewhere between Fredericksburg and Chancellorsville."

"As we don't know where the battles will be fought," Heath asked, "do we have other plantations, churches, or farmhouses that might serve as general hospitals?"

Pointing to the Romain's hospital on the map, Guild said, "This one is the furthest west. No one knows where the battle will be, so I'm guessing the two hospitals furthest from the battle will need to relocate."

"Supplies?" Simon asked.

Guild replied, "The quartermaster will send messengers to each general hospital each morning to see what is needed."

"Dr. Heath and Dr. Jordan," Rachel interrupted, "do you know what we're asking of you regarding our research?"

"Not exactly," Clerk said, "Can't say I care much. When injured men start arriving in numbers, we'll not have the time nor the inclination to do anything but operate."

"We ask only that you keep records on men who need amputation within forty-eight hours of injury. After surgery, our patients with amputations will need to be put together in specific tents away from others. Nothing more," Simon said. "Date of injury, type of surgery, and outcome."

"You think you're better than us and trying to prove it," Heath spit out a vindictive, his neck veins bulging and both hands in a fist. "Fancy language, red-coat training means nothing. When you've been up for thirty-six hours without time to take a piss, we'll see how you do. Simon, you might last ten, twelve hours. Your pretty niece here won't last five before she faints and needs a nap."

"John, watch your manners," Guild said. "That was uncalled for until we see how they perform."

"I'll last, you fat swab," Rachel snapped back, holding her composure as best she could. "You try and stay on deck in the Indian Ocean during a typhoon for thirty-six hours straight. So knackered you can't feel your fingers or toes. I've done it. You couldn't."

Heath stood and started walking toward Rachel. Guild jumped up between Rachel and Heath.

"I have no damn idea what you're talking about, Miss," Heath yelled over Guild's shoulder, "except that you shouldn't be here. You're no better than a damn Yankee."

Simon grabbed Rachel's forearm. The room became deadly quiet.

"We're working together," Guild said. "Don't need you fighting when there's work to be done. We'll all do our best. As with previous battles, we will treat any Yankee injury after all our injuries have been dealt with."

"I won't treat 'em," Heath said.

"I, for one," Rachel said, "will not refuse to treat any human who might benefit. It's unconscionable not to. Send us those men."

"I agree," Simon said.

"We don't see that many Yankees," Guild said, "so it's not a big deal. Their doctors do the same for our men."

"Each of you have support staff," Simon said. "We've only us two plus two slaves we purchased in Richmond. Dr. Moore said we're on our own but if we're overwhelmed, we'll need help."

Heath scowled but held his tongue.

"I won't promise anything until I see how you do," Guild said. "If you're productive, I can give you men. You've got a big house to work with."

"Thank you," Rachel said.

Simon added, "Both of our slaves have manumission

papers and after the war, they will be sent to Chicago. Because we were provided no assistance, both have been taught to enter data. They are not to be punished."

"Damn Yankees," Heath mumbled.

That night, assuming the worst, Simon and Rachel agreed that Bessy and Flora might be needed to give anesthesia if either Rachel or Simon needed a surgical assistant for complicated procedures. Using freshly made masks for the ether or chloroform, the two slaves practiced holding the masks on Simon, Rachel and each other.

"Simon or I will tell you whilst you hold the masks how much to drip. Chloroform is much stronger than ether. Ether might catch fire so it can't be used at night when we need lanterns and candles for light. It will depend on what's available."

"Never heard no such thing as 'ether,' or dat 'chloro' stuff," Bessy said. "I'll believes it whens I sees it."

At dawn on May 1, the sounds of artillery disturbed an otherwise peaceful morning[17]. An hour later, the first

---

[17] *Background – Battle of Chancellorsville*

From the onset of the Civil War in July 1861, the Union Army of the Potomac had one failure after another, despite having more men and armament than the Army of North Virginia. At the end of 1862, the morale of the Army of Potomac had fallen to its lowest point.

In January 1863, Abraham Lincoln appointed General Joe Hooker as the new commander of the Union's Army of the Potomac.

Hooker brimmed with confidence and spent the winter months of 1863 revitalizing his army and instilling new confidence. By April, Hooker believed his army and plans were ready to take on Robert E. Lee and the Army of North Virginia.

Hooker boasted to any who would listen, "I have the finest army on the planet. I have the finest army the sun ever shone on. If the enemy does not run, God help them. May God have mercy on General Lee, for I will have none."

On April 27, 1863, Hooker and the Army of the Potomac forded the Rappahannock River west of Fredericksburg. The next day, as part of Hooker's master plan, Major General George Stoneman, Jr., led the Army of the Potomac's cavalry and crossed the Rappahannock River west of the small village of Chancellorsville.

ambulance arrived at the Romains' hospital with two injured men. One soldier's scalp had been grazed by a bullet. Rachel, with Bessy's help, cleaned the wound and sutured it closed. The man returned to the frontlines three hours later. Another man had an open fracture of his lower right leg inches above the ankle. Both tibia and fibula were shattered and a good portion of skin was missing from the lower calf.

Heavily sedated with morphine and opium gum, the man raised his head and asked, "I'm gonna lose my leg, ain't I?"

Simon said, "Yes. There is no other choice. The lower leg is gone."

Simon scrubbed his hands while Rachel proceeded to drip chloroform into the gauze mask covering the man's nose and mouth. Bessy cut away the remnants of the man's leggings. When Simon made an incision circumferentially around the man's calf, above the injury, Flora covered her mouth.

"I's gonna be sick," she cried, then ran out of the house.

Rachel shook her head. "Bessy, you'll need to talk to your daughter. We need her. There will be more of this, plus cleaning to do."

"I'll talk to her," Bessy said. "She ain't never skinned

Stoneman headed south toward Hanover Junction to attack Lee's supply lines. By doing so, he lost contact with Hooker's army.

Hooker expected Stoneman's raid to draw Lee away to protect Richmond, but the ruse didn't work as Lee refused to engage Stoneman. Stoneman's departure also allowed Lee's cavalry under J.E.B. 'Jeb' Stuart to move unhindered around Hooker's army.

Hooker and his army then crossed the Rapidan River and set up lines east of an area called the 'Wilderness of Spotsylvania,' commonly known only as the 'Wilderness,' a densely forested area of second-growth trees.

On May 1, 1863, Hooker exited the Wilderness and marched toward Lee, believing, erroneously, the Confederates would be divided and busy on two fronts.

a chicken or slaughtered a hog."

"Come here and hold the chloroform mask, please. We'll tell you when to drip more like we showed you," Rachel said as Simon applied a tourniquet above the knee. Minutes later, Rachel, hands scrubbed in dilute sodium hypochlorite, came to assist.

Twenty minutes later, Rachel said, "Bessy, take off the mask. We're almost done. Hold his head and chin back like I showed you so he can breathe fresh air."

As cannon fire boomed in the background, the stump of this first amputation was bandaged and the man transferred to a stretcher and taken outside by Simon and Flora where he was laid on the ground.

"Not bad for a first case," Simon said, as Rachel sat with Bessy helping her enter the first patient into their logbook.

"I wonder if we've under or overestimated the number of assistants we'll need," Rachel said. "If it gets busy, we could use another surgeon and three qualified assistants to give anesthesia plus some aides."

"Maybe, maybe not," Simon said. "Let's see if we get busy."

As they wrote, Flora ran back into the house and yelled, "There be ten wagons coming up the road."

The first three injured men were carried into the house. The rest of the ambulances emptied their men, thirty-eight in all, onto the lawn and porch in front of the house. The ambulances then turned back toward the cannon fire.

Rachel directed the stretcher bearers into the five operating theaters as Lafayette Guild ran into the house with six men trailing him.

"Your hospital is the closest to the front," Guild cried. "You can't possibly handle all this."

"We need more help," Rachel shouted, already focusing. "Another four surgeons, and six who can give chloroform or ether, and ten aides or nurses."

"You'll need even more than that! My hospital is the

furthest from the front and will be underserved. I've shut it down and we'll stay with you. Four of these men can give the anesthetic, if needed. I have my full cadre of surgeons and assistants on the way. We'll set up general hospitals in tents and other rooms."

"That should work," Simon said.

"Don't count on me to scrub my hands, instruments and sheets," Guild said.

We don't expect you to, but we still need aides," Rachel said.

"I'll send a man to find you another ten," Guild said.

The cacophony of mixed sounds would permeate the hospital for the next three days and nights – booming cannons afar mixed with the screams of pain, yells for help, gasping for air of agonal patients about to die, and pleas to their mothers, wives and God.

Twelve medics arrived soon thereafter. Those ten helped Guild and Simon, while Rachel asked that Bessy and Flora stay with her as she could count on them to scrub their hands. Guild gave Rachel a first-year medical student from New Orleans, William Fleischman, who had no experience with anesthesia.

Rachel told Fleischmann that Bessy and Flora were her slaves and she expected him to treat them kindly. "Bessy will show you how to hold and apply the masks. I will tell you how much to drip depending on which anesthetic you use."

Fleischmann and Bessy worked together for most of the morning and early afternoon until Fleischmann felt comfortable holding the anesthesia masks by himself, although he never thanked Bessy for the lessons.

As quickly as one patient received treatment of any kind, the surgeon would yell, "Stretcher!" Only Simon and Rachel would specify to the stretcher bearers that their amputees would be placed in specific tents.

Aides appeared and the patients whisked away in

seconds, to be replaced by another injured soldier. Treated and untreated men covered every inch of ground around the converted farmhouse.

Throughout the night and early morning, Guild, Simon, Rachel, and the other surgeons barely saw one another, except for the occasional thirty second consultation, always about whether a patient could be saved or the level of amputation to be done. Long past nightfall, the sound of cannon quieted and Heath's relocated general hospital became functional, alleviating much of the congestion. The last ambulance of injured men arrived in the early hours of the morning.

Simon and Rachel, both exhausted, sat against the wall in the house's dining room, the largest of six operating theaters. They sat despite the blood that caked the wooden floor and dotted the wallpaper and ceiling. There were speckles of blood on their hair, face, neck and uniforms. The heavy odor of old blood and sweat hung in the air; it would permeate the house for months after they had departed.

Rachel moistened her lips with her tongue, spitting specks of blood. "My hands ache from the scrubs," she said. "I don't know if we can dilute it further."

"We can't change the formula until we've done enough patients," Simon said.

"I know," Rachel said. "Too bad."

"I never could've imagined this would be as terrible as it was," Simon said, "and I've never been so tired."

"At least with a nightmare, you awaken and it's gone. This nightmare will keep coming, over and over," Rachel sighed.

"Did you see the numbers?" Simon asked.

"Yes. Twenty-eight amputations logged between us," she said. "Six arms above the elbow, two below, fifteen below the knee and five above the knee. Guild and the others had one hundred-four amputations."

"Sobering," Simon said. "I had at least twenty men come in too far gone to save. Another fifteen had massive chest or abdominal injuries. I gave them enough morphine to make them comfortable until they died. They knew when they arrived that we could do nothing for them. That was the most disconcerting thing."

Rachel sniffled and nodded. She'd seen men in that condition too.

Guild walked into the room looking every bit as exhausted.

"Sit," Rachel said. "I've sent Bessy and Flora up to their room to sleep. When I have enough energy to stand, I'll join them."

Guild nodded but remained standing. "I was wrong about both of you," he said. "I came in a few times and watched you work. You came prepared and your techniques are flawless."

"Thank you," Simon said.

"I still don't believe in scrubbing with hypochlorite," Guild said. "I think it a waste of time but I don't see how it hurts."

"Even if hypochlorite doesn't work, we've still have proven something," Rachel said.

Guild laughed. "Well, then you'd have made a huge trip at great expense for nothing."

"Some things need proving or disproving," Rachel repeated.

"Yes." Guild shook his head as he looked at her and said, "I suppose. You are different from any woman I've ever met."

"I'll take that as a compliment."

"It was meant that way."

"I would kill for a bath," Rachel said.

"Not yet. Perhaps, just a change of clothing. We all need sleep. I sent all the other surgeons and assistants to bed. Tomorrow could be worse." Without another word, Guild went outside to his tent.

Simon helped Rachel up and they started to climb the narrow stairs to their bedrooms.

"He's not so bad, I guess," Rachel said.

"From the sound of it, he's already been to hell and back," Simon said. "I'm glad he's here and in charge."

Just then, Guild re-entered the house and called to Rachel and Simon.

"Forgot to mention, there's a Yankee officer who's been here for half a day. Shot in the arm somewhere. Feel free to look at him. The sentry outside knows where they put him. It's dark and a few men are drunk out there, so if Rachel goes, take a sentry with you. I shouldn't have to tell you why." Guild didn't wait for a reply before leaving.

Rachel turned to Simon and said, "I'll go. I don't know if I can sleep yet."

She headed down the stairs and asked one of the two sentries stationed outside the door where the injured Yankee prisoners might be.

"There be two bluebellies[18] in the last tent down the last row," the sentry said, pointing past the row of tents. "Not that I gives a damn, but someone told me one of thems is dead as a doornail."

Rachel said, "You'll need to escort me there."

The other sentry said, "We ain't s'posed to leave our post, Ma'am."

"Orders from Colonel Guild are that I be escorted," Rachel said. "If I have to wake the colonel to repeat the order, I'm pretty sure both of you will be cleaning sink holes[19] for a month."

The sentries looked at each other and shrugged.

"This way, Ma'am," the first sentry said.

Rachel walked past rows of large tents housing up to ten injured men each. The moans of post-operative patients captured the night air. At the last tent on the furthest row, she saw a guard asleep at the opening. She tapped

---

[18] During the Civil War, Union soldiers were called "bluebellies" by the Confederates. The Union soldiers called the Confederates, "graybacks."

[19] Sink holes or sinks: dugout trenches used for refuse and garbage.

him on the shoulder and he jumped awake and reached for his rifle.

"Sorry, Ma'am. Musta dozed off. Didn't hear nuttin' inside this bluebelly tent," the guard said.

"I'm a surgeon and Colonel Guild thought I should look in. Is it okay to enter?" Rachel asked.

"Fine by me. One of 'em's been dead for a spell I s'pose. Other one at the far end is probably asleep 'cause, like I said, I ain't heard nuttin'. Here's a lantern, 'cause it's awful dark in there."

Holding the lantern, Rachel entered the tent, which was dimly lit with four candles in each corner. To her right, she saw a body covered with a sheet. She picked up the sheet and raised her lantern to find a dead Union soldier with a gaping wound of his chest and abdomen.

Replacing the sheet, she walked to the far end of the tent to find a man asleep on the ground with crude, blood-soaked bandages around his left hand. He wore the uniform of a Union captain, a navy-blue long coat and sky-blue trousers. On his shoulders sat sewn-on epaulets with two gold bars denoting his rank. She nudged him until he opened his eyes.

"Hello. Hello, I'm Dr. Rachel Romain. I'd like to look at your injury."

The officer grimaced when he tried to use his injured hand to sit up. He quickly switched to his right hand. "Thank you. I thought no one would ever come."

Rachel raised her lantern and took a close look at the man. Looking past his dirty face, she thought him handsome with fair skin, soft brown eyes, thick, wavy auburn hair, and two days' worth of stubble.

"Do you have any other injuries?" she asked.

"No, just my hand and a bruised shoulder. I fell off my wagon after being shot."

"When were you shot?"

"Yesterday morning, about eleven. For that matter, what day is it? I've lost track of time."

"It's about 3 a.m., Saturday morning," Rachel said.

"Come with me back to the hospital where I can get a better look at it. What's your name?"

Still disoriented, the officer mumbled, "Hmmph. It's still the Sabbath." He had trouble getting up with one good hand.

"I asked your name," Rachel said as she helped him stand. She looked surprised at his height, a full head above hers.

"Thank you, Ma'am. Solomon Birch. Quartermaster, First New York Brigade."

"Nice to meet you, Solomon Birch," Rachel said. "What happened?"

"I took the wrong turn trying to bring ammunition to the front. Are you English?"

"Yes, from London. Stay here so I can tell the guard I'm taking you to the hospital."

In the hospital, Rachel lit extra lanterns for light. Solomon sat with his hand on the table as she unwrapped his blood-soaked bandages.

His little finger was gone and half the ring finger from the middle knuckle out remained attached by only a sliver of skin.

"Oh my," Solomon said, eyes wide open. "It's the first I've looked at it."

"Could've been worse. Much worse," Rachel said. "I'll need to remove the dangling half of the unattached ring finger and clean up the little finger wound."

"Are you a surgeon?" Solomon asked.

"Yes, I'm a surgeon."

"How unusual. A young, beautiful, woman surgeon. I'll bet there's a story behind that," Solomon said.

Rachel nodded, "Yes. A rather long one. No time for that now. Maybe in the morning."

"Will it hurt, what you're planning to do?"

"Quite a bit," Rachel said, "for about fifteen minutes, unless I have you put to sleep with chloroform."

"You can do both at the same time?" Solomon asked.

"No. I'll need to awaken my aide who can do the anesthetic."

"I'd like that. Thank you."

"I'm curious," Rachel said. "In your tent, you said it was the Sabbath. It's not Sunday yet."

"I'm Jewish," Solomon said. "Different Sabbath."

Rachel smiled. "I assumed so. Did you light Sabbath candles last night?"

"No, of course I didn't," Solomon said. "I was watching another man die. It was ghastly hearing him take his last breaths." He hesitated. "Why do you ask? That's a strange question coming from most anyone around here."

"I suppose it is," she said.

Confused, Simon watched as she blew out one of the lit candles and put it between them. She took a clean towel from her pocket and put it over her head, then took a nearby lit candle and re-lit the one she had already blown out.

"Ready," she said as she closed her eyes and waved both hands over the newly lit candle. "*Baruch Atah Adonai...*"

Solomon, flabbergasted as Rachel began chanting the Sabbath prayer in Hebrew, joined in.

"*Eloheinu Melech halolam. Asher kid'shanu b'mitzvotav v'zivanu l'hadlik ner shel Shabbat.*"

Solomon smiled. "In a million years, I would have never guessed. If I live through this war, no one will believe I was rescued by a young, beautiful, British, Jewish, female surgeon who said the Sabbath prayer with me."

"I wouldn't believe it either," Rachel laughed.

Solomon's eyes fell on Andrew's engagement ring, which Rachel always wore.

"You're married," he said.

"Ah, no. Almost – engaged some time ago to a soldier. He passed before we wed," Rachel said. "Another story I don't have time to tell."

"I'm sorry. May his memory be for a blessing."

"Thank you. Anyway, stay here. My anesthetist is a black female slave I purchased in Richmond. So don't act too surprised."

Solomon's face grew rigid.

"Ah," he said. "You own slaves."

"Yes," Rachel said. "I bought two, mother and daughter, to keep them from being sold apart. My uncle and I are here to do research. The North refused our request, so we came to the South. I needed assistants and the Confederacy offered none."

"Still, you bought slaves, no matter the reason," Solomon said with a grimace.

Rachel shook her head. "You misunderstand. I deplore the thought of slavery. It is evil beyond comprehension and has been rightfully outlawed everywhere in the British empire for more than three decades. I've already given manumission papers to both mother and daughter. They will stay with me as long as I work in the South and are being paid a fair salary. I've promised them that I will not let them be separated or put back in slavery."

"I feel better hearing that," Solomon said.

"We must proceed," Rachel said. "I'll put some laudanum vials in your trouser pockets in case the pain is too much and will check on you in the morning. I doubt anyone here will offer you anything to eat, so I'll add a few biscuits as well. That's all I have to give. Your hand will feel better if you keep it elevated."

"Thank you. I wish I was meeting you under different circumstances."

"Perhaps we'll meet again and share stories."

"I hope so," Solomon said.

Rachel ran upstairs to awaken Bessy. Twenty-five minutes later, Solomon's wound was dressed and he was carted back to his tent by two soldiers.

The next morning, cannon fire again awakened Simon

and Rachel at dawn[20]. Rachel had two hours of sleep, Simon three. She told Simon the story of Solomon Birch and added, "I don't know why and it makes no sense, but it's the first time since Andrew that I liked someone from the beginning. There's something there. I'd like to get to know him."

"I'm afraid," Simon said, "you've little time for that."

When Rachel and Simon came downstairs, Lafayette Guild was waiting.

"Stonewall left early this morning with thirty thousand men, trying to outflank Hooker," Guild said. "It's going to be bloody. I hope you're ready."

"We're ready," Rachel said. "First, I want to check on someone."

She grabbed bandages, a few vials of laudanum, a cup of cold coffee, and a slice of buttered bread, then headed out the door to see how Solomon had fared.

Solomon, awake, sat up as soon as Rachel entered the tent.

"How are you feeling this morning?" Rachel asked.

"It hurts," Solomon said, "but, as you said, it's better when I keep it elevated. I slept well with the laudanum. Thank you."

"You're welcome. You'll have pain for another day, then you'll feel much better," Rachel said. "I've brought some more laudanum for you. Keep it hidden, as the guards will take it. Also some buttered bread. I'm

---

[20] *Background Battle of Chancellorsville – Day Two*
Despite having the high ground and more numbers, General Hooker wasn't prepared for the aggressive actions of Lee. Hooker decided to retreat into the Wilderness to fight a defensive battle. Hooker's generals couldn't understand this error in judgment and most historians agree this battle was lost on that decision. Jeb Stuart's cavalry, having free rein with the North's Cavalry absent, discovered Hooker's right flank was poorly defended. Lee and his second in command, Stonewall Jackson, would use this weakness to their advantage.

guessing they haven't fed you."

"Thank you," Solomon said.

Rachel undid the bandages and examined the wounds. "Looks good."

As she rebandaged his hand, Solomon watched Rachel's face.

"You are a special person, I think. A remarkable woman of valor," he said. "I doubt anyone else would have come to look at my hand."

"Unfortunately, you're probably right," Rachel said as she finished. "Are you a career soldier?"

"No, never, ever," Solomon said.

"Good," Rachel said, "I've sad memories of career soldiers."

"As you said last night. I studied philosophy and logic at Harvard College, hoping to teach," Solomon said, "but ended up in the family business. My family works in metals, making kitchen utensils, like knives and forks and such. All started by my grandfather years ago."

"I believe I am logical," Rachel said, "but I know nothing of philosophy and you know little of medicine. You should consider making surgical instruments. Then we'd have much to talk about."

"I'd seriously consider it if it meant seeing you again," Solomon said, smiling. "You were going to tell me how you got into surgery."

"You'd have to hear my entire story to make sense of it all. I'm here only to do research on preventing infection in wounds after surgery using chlorine scrubbing. An obstetrician in Hungary has eradicated infection after childbirth. I'm here to use his techniques on amputation."

"It's as if you're speaking a foreign tongue," Solomon said.

"Fine, what do you do when you're not making forks and spoons?"

"My family owns a vacation home on Cape Cod, a long peninsula not far from Boston. I sail whenever there. Have you ever been sailing? Other than your voyage here, I suppose."

Rachel laughed. "More than you'd believe, but I've got to return to the hospital now. We're expecting casualties all day and into the night."

"Will you promise to return?" Solomon asked. "I'd love to talk more."

"Most definitely."

"As I said last night, I wish we'd met under different circumstances. You may be the only good thing that has happened to me during this hellish war."

"I'll be back. I promise."

"What will happen to me here? Do you know?" Solomon asked.

"I assume they will put you in a prison camp," Rachel said.

Solomon shuddered.

"We've all heard stories about the Confederate camps. None too nice, with little food or shelter. Many die of disease or starvation. I'm guessing then I'll never see you again to hear the story of why you're a surgeon. I would have loved to hear it all."

"I know nothing of the camps," Rachel said, "but the soldiers here are already short on food and clothing. I imagine the prisoners are much worse. If I could hide you, I would. For now, I'll tell the guard you're not ready to leave for another couple of days. I can't promise they'll listen."

"If nothing else, it was nice meeting you, Rachel Romain," Solomon said. "I believe that fate had us meeting for some bigger purpose."

"Likewise Solomon Birch," Rachel said. She extended her right hand for him to shake but Solomon took firm hold of her hand and stood. With tears at the edge of his eyelids, he kissed her hand and said, "Thank you for everything."

Solomon tried to release her hand but Rachel kept it near to his lips. She looked up at him, transfixed by his tears and his fears of what was to come in a Confederate prison. She leaned closer and kissed him on the cheek.

Separating, she said, "I do hope we can spend time together before you're sent away. I'll come again tonight when free."

Back in the hospital, Rachel told Simon about Solomon.

"You like him," Solomon asked.

"I do. Very much so after such a short time. His family sails," she said.

"You know he'll be sent away," Simon said. "You won't be able to see him again until the end of this ridiculous war."

"And I've not had good luck with men in the army."

Simon nodded but said nothing.

Rachel, Simon and the other surgeons worked without stopping from 8 a.m. to 6 p.m. The ambulances were lined up as far as the eye could see. Rachel told Guild she needed to eat something.

"Don't spend too long," Guild said. "But I don't need to tell you."

Rachel grabbed a piece of cold mutton and a slice of bread to share with Solomon and headed out to his tent. No guard stood watch and inside she found only the dead Union soldier. Worried, she found a nearby sentry and asked what had happened to Solomon.

"Some officers picked him up 'bout an hour ago," the soldier said.

Rachel gasped, "Oh, no. He's not going to be hurt, is he?"

"Not sure 'bout that," the soldier replied with a shrug. "I think I heard tell he was bein' swapped for one of our captured generals."

Shaking her head at the strangeness of the past day, Rachel took a bite of the mutton as she hurried back to the hospital.

Rachel, Simon, and Guild worked non-stop until the

line of ambulances dwindled. Guild departed on horseback after telling Simon and Rachel they could handle the rest of the injured soldiers and that he needed to check on Heath and Clerk.

At 9 p.m., a large group of Confederate cavalry arrived along with an ambulance. Two officers ran into the house screaming, "Where are the surgeons? Where are the surgeons?"

Simon and an aide were finishing an arm amputation, so Rachel met the officers at the door.

"What's happening?" Rachel asked. "I'm a surgeon."

"We need a real surgeon," the lead officer said.

"I am a real surgeon," Rachel said. "Tell me what's happening."

"General Jackson has been shot," the next officer said. "He's lost a lot of blood."

A few seconds later, the men carried General Thomas 'Stonewall' Jackson into the house and laid him on the table in front of Rachel. Rachel saw considerable blood soaking the general's left arm and wrist and the right hand. Five officers now surrounded Jackson.

"Cut off his jacket and shirt," Rachel commanded, "so we can see the extent of the injuries." As an officer cut away Jackson's clothing, Rachel screamed, "I need room to work. I need the rest of you men to stand back or leave."

One of the officers asked, "When will the senior surgeons arrive?"

"I am a surgeon. You'll have to trust me," Rachel said. "Move back."

The idle officers, all unable to hold back tears, moved away to the wall of the room to watch.

Once the coat and shirt had been cut away, Rachel could see blood oozing from the wound below an ineffective tourniquet high on the left arm. She replaced the tourniquet just under the shoulder, which stopped the bleeding. Simon, done with his case, entered the room to assist.

"Thank God, a real surgeon," another officer declared.

Rachel could only shake her head.

"You men should only be so lucky to have Dr. Romain take care of you if injured," Simon barked. Turning to Rachel, he said, "I'm sorry. Who is the patient?"

"Some general," Rachel said.

An officer's voice came from behind Simon. "That's Stonewall Jackson, Lee's second in command."

"General Jackson, Dr. Romain and I are here to take care of you," Simon said. Simon inspected the left arm wounds and the right palm. "General, you've shattered your left upper arm and wrist. The right palm wound is superficial and will heal on its own. We need to remove the left arm below the shoulder. Do you understand?"

Jackson, heavily sedated with laudanum, whispered, "Yes. Do what you must."

As Rachel started the chloroform anesthetic, Simon went to scrub his hands with hypochlorite. One of Guild's anesthetists entered and Rachel let him take over the anesthesia so she could scrub her hands. As she scrubbed, Lafayette Guild ran into the house with another man, Dr. Hunter McGuire, Stonewall Jackson's personal physician.

"Is it true General Jackson has been shot?" Guild cried.

"I'm afraid so," Rachel said.

"Dr. McGuire and I must assist," Guild said. Without scrubbing, McGuire and Guild approached Simon, who handed the scalpel to the Confederate surgeons.

"The case is yours," Simon said.

At the same time, Rachel relieved the anesthetist.

Twenty-five minutes later, bandages encased Jackson's stump and shoulder as Rachel allowed Jackson to awaken.

"We'll find a nearby house for him to recover," McGuire said. "It is a dark day, indeed. General Lee will be lost without him."

Once awake, Jackson's officers carried him out to a waiting ambulance.

At last, quiet surrounded the hospital.

"I'm sorry the men did not treat you as a surgeon," Simon said.

"They didn't know," Rachel said, shrugging. "I'm an odd duck, remember."

"But a competent odd-duck. Do you know our numbers?" Simon asked.

"Bessy thinks we've reached ninety cases," Rachel said. "Guild and the other surgeons have over two hundred. We've one infection so far. The other surgeons have eleven."

As Rachel had feared, the other surgeons were failing to keep records of their procedures. She decided that she and Bessy would need to make rounds on the other injured amputees as well.

At six-thirty the following morning, the third day of fighting resumed.[21] Simon, Rachel, Guild and the rest of the men stood at the house's entrance, awaiting the ambulances sure to come.

John Heath limped into the house and approached Guild.

"John, why are you here?" Guild asks. "All hell's

---

[21] *Background – Battle of Chancellorsville – Day 3*

After his amputation, Stonewall Jackson was transported to a nearby plantation in Guiney Station, Virginia. Jackson had been shot by his own men, believing he and his entourage to be Union soldiers. 'Stonewall' Jackson would die eight days later from pneumonia.

The next day, May 3rd, the armies lined up against each other at the edge of the Wilderness. With the brutal fighting, injuries mounted on each side. Hooker again showed his reluctance to fight and retreated deeper into the Wilderness. A Union rear guard attack from the east required Lee to divide his army to hold the Union army at bay.

about to break loose."

"My gout's acting up. I can't stand," Heath said. "There'll be no senior surgeon at my General Hospital."

"So much for outlasting me," Rachel said.

Heath sneered at Rachel, to little effect.

"I could send Miss Romain to relieve you for the day," Guild said.

"She's not a surgeon. Send her uncle if you must."

Guild replied without hesitation. "You're wrong, John. She's quite good and lasts as long as the rest of us. More experienced than you and most others, I'm afraid."

Heath, disbelieving Guild's comment, looked to the other assistants who either looked away or nodded agreement with Guild.

"We'd rather stay together," Simon said, "to continue our research."

"Then I'll have to go myself," Guild said with a grimace of disgust.

Rachel looked at Guild and said, "As much as I hate relieving Dr. Heath of his discomfort, you might suggest taking colchicine for the gout if he can handle the stomach upset."

"I don't need your foolish advice," Heath snapped at Rachel's back and limped toward her.

While Guild looked daggers at Rachel, Simon stood firmly between the two combatants. Rachel knew she'd taken her tone and comment a step too far said over Simon's shoulder, "Sorry, John."

Guild gathered his surgical tools and headed for the door with a hobbled Heath.

"No matter how much evidence you show some people, you cannot convince an idiot," Rachel said loud enough to be heard.

Heath started to turn back to Rachel but Guild pushed him forward out the door.

When the men were out of earshot, Simon said, "My dear niece, I wish Cynthia were here to help you work on your people skills. They seem to be lacking. We are guests of this government and they could ask us to leave before we have the chance to finish our research."

"That man riles me so," Rachel said.

"If it's any comfort," Simon said, "I believe he riles Lafayette as well."

The ambulances with injured and dying men came all day and night. The cannon fire ended at sundown, but the ambulances kept coming until 10 p.m. The surgeries lasted until 2 a.m. Rachel and Bessy stayed up an extra hour tallying the surgeries and making rounds on all the men operated on by both teams.

In the morning, Rachel read the tallies to Simon.

"One hundred-five for you and me, about equal number of leg and arm amputations. Four-hundred for Guild and the others that we know of. We have three known infections which required re-amputation. Six possible we're watching."

"We're half way to our goal of two hundred," Simon said.

"We don't know if the other general hospitals are keeping tabs or not, or if they'd be honest. Here, Guild and his men have needed to re-amputate twenty-six already and have had one death."

"Sounds favorable," Simon said. "Do the other surgeons know our numbers?"

"I thought it best not to tell them," Rachel said. "As far as they know we're doing about the same. Our guards and assistants have an inkling as to how we're doing. Two of the men have come up to me and said they'd want you or me taking care of them if injured."

Simon said, "I've had the same conversations with the men. They know. I've told them they must not talk of it."

"Hard not to, I'd think," Rachel said.

On May 4th, segments of Lee's divided army repelled the

Union rear guard around Fredericksburg and forced them back across the Rappahannock River. For Rachel and Simon, the battle near Chancellorsville was relatively quiet, with ambulances arriving only until 2 p.m. The surgeries were completed by 6 p.m. For the first time in four days, the surgeons, including Simon and Rachel, had a sit-down dinner and got to sleep by 10 p.m.

The following day, fighting ceased and Hooker and the Army of the Potomac crossed back over the Rappahannock River to head north toward Washington. The Army of the Potomac started with ninety-seven thousand men while Lee started with fifty-seven thousand men. Combined North and South, the Battle of Chancellorsville had more than thirteen thousand injured, dead or missing.

A day after the Union retreat, Simon complained that he felt feverish,[22] suffering from a headache and stomach upset. Each day his symptoms worsened and he took to bed. Meanwhile, Rachel, Guild, Heath, Clerk and the rest of the Confederate Medical Corps spent the ensuing week treating the men injured in battle. At the same time, Rachel and Bessy tallied their results and those of the other surgeons.

As Rachel, Bessy and Flora began packing their equipment, Simon took a turn for the worse. He had a high fever, severe stomach pain, shortness of breath, bloody diarrhea and generalized weakness. Guild, Heath, Clerk and Rachel conferred and all agreed that Simon had contracted typhoid fever.

While the four surgeons agreed on a diagnosis, they disagreed on treatment. Heath thought bloodletting might rid Simon of his 'evil' humors, Clerk wanted to use turpentine, and Guild favored quinine. Rachel wanted only to treat his known symptoms with bed rest and opiates for the loose stools. In the end, the other

[22] Thomas Allbutt (1836–1925) devised the first small clinical thermometer in 1867. Fever, before then, was a clinical guess.

physicians deferred to Rachel. Simon was placed in the back of an army ambulance and transported slowly back to Richmond with Flora beside him.

The same day, Rachel and Bessy headed by wagon back to Richmond as well, arriving a day earlier than Simon's ambulance. Rachel secured the same house they'd rented a month earlier and waited for Simon and Flora to arrive the next morning. Over the next week, Simon languished in bed with stomach discomfort, remaining weak and disoriented at times. Rachel guessed he had lost twenty pounds from his normal weight of one-hundred-fifty. A week later, under Rachel and Bessie's care, Simon showed signs of improvement. His fevers disappeared and he tolerated small amounts of bland food without increasing his stomach discomfort or having diarrhea.

Guild came to visit and validated Rachel's regimen of bland food and opiates.

"We've won the battle at Chancellorsville," Guild said. "Lee thinks it's time to head north, defeat the Army of Potomac once and for all, and take Washington. He thinks the North will then be forced to sue for peace."

"Why are you telling me this?" Rachel asked.

"Generals Ewell and Stuart have asked for you and your father's services by name when they head north. They don't know of Simon's illness," Guild said. "I'd also be joining you."

"Heath?" Rachel asked.

"No. His gout is still problematic. That should make you happy," Guild said. "Clerk had to return to Atlanta."

"I wouldn't mind Heath if only he could show me an ounce of respect," Rachel said. "Let me talk to Simon. I hate to leave him, but I also know he wants us to finish our research."

Simon, seemingly on the mend, implored Rachel to leave with Guild. On June 5th, 1863, Rachel and Bessy headed north to the site of Jeb Stuart's cavalry encampment. Bessy agreed that Flora should remain in

Richmond to care for Simon.

On June 7th, Rachel and Bessy arrived in Brandy Station, a small village thirty-two miles northeast from Fredericksburg. The area bustled with energy with Jeb Stuart's cavalry having nine thousand cavalry and four batteries of horse artillery. Rachel asked directions from some sentries and found Lafayette Guild outside a vacant church south of the Brandy Station.

"This building will easily hold six operating tables and has ample storage," Guild said. "I've left everything in crates, thinking we'll need to move when Stuart heads north in front of Lcc's army."

"What do we do now?" Rachel asked.

"Sit tight and wait. We often move on short notice."

Rachel and Guild did not have to wait long; the Union Cavalry of the Army of the Potomac launched a surprise attack on Stuart's Cavalry on the morning of June 9th at 4:30 in the morning. The one-day battle lasted until 10 p.m. and ended with the Union withdrawing back over the Rappahannock River.

Rachel, Guild and the other surgeons worked all day and most of the next, treating injured soldiers. Rachel and Bessy stayed near Brandy Station for the next week, compiling data on her surgical outcomes with hypochlorite scrubbing, versus those of the other surgeons.

Once completing their survey, Rachel and Bessy returned to Richmond to visit Simon, who remained sick with intermittent fevers and diarrhea. His skin, the color of dirty ash and dotted with small rose spots was taut over his thin frame like a rope-tension-snare-drum head used by marching soldiers. On the positive side, he'd lost no more weight and had tolerated broths and bland food.

"You must return," Simon said, "and finish our work now that we're so close to the finish line. We need just two hundred cases."

"Damn the research. I should be with you. If something were to happen, Mum would never forgive me."

"With Flora's care, I'm improving day by day. And if you don't finish the research. I'll never forgive you nor will you forgive yourself. This was your endeavor first. I'm too weak to argue. Go."

The next day Rachel and Bessy headed back north to find Lee's army heading north toward the Potomac River, Maryland and Pennsylvania.

On the wagon heading north, Rachel repeated her fear over leaving Simon to Bessy.

"I swore to my mum," Rachel said, "that I wouldn't leave Simon. But I've done it. God help me if something happens to him."

Bessy consoled Rachel as best she could. "He be fine and there ain't nuttin' more you can do but just watch him. Simon be a doctor too. Flora will take good care of him and will do whatever he ask of her."

"If nothing else, Bessy, you need to keep telling me he'll be okay or I'll lose my mind."

"He be fine."

Chapter Sixteen
1863 Gettysburg

General Robert E. Lee dismounted Traveller, his magnificent 16-hand[23] American Saddlebred gray stallion, and handed the reins to a waiting Confederate soldier. He had just arrived at his headquarters north of the Potomac River. Approaching his command tent, Lee found Rachel in the white-collared outfit of a nurse and a large, face-covering sun hat. She stood beside two armed sentinels of the Army of North Virginia. She had never seen Lee before. He appeared to be a normal person, taller than most and well-groomed but not the God everyone made him out to be.

Both guards snapped to attention and the senior sentry, a corporal, spoke. "Sir. General Stuart been in your tent for 'bout an hour 'waiting fer you gettin' here." The guard turned his head toward Rachel and added, "This lady said you wanted to speak to her."

"Thank you, Corporal," Lee said, then addressed Rachel. "I do need to speak with you. Do you mind waiting for a short spell? Army business."

Unaccustomed to army protocols, Rachel shrugged acceptance, said nothing, and found a seat on a small tree stump nearby.

Lee entered the tent to find his favorite cavalry officer, Jeb Stuart, lying on a cot in a deep sleep. Lee nudged Stuart's shoulder, which startled the dreaming officer awake. Stuart sat up and reached for his revolver. He came quickly to his senses and smiled.

"Sorry 'bout that, Robert," he said, yawning.

"It's okay. You need your rest," Lee said. "Thanks for not shooting me. Are you awake enough for orders?"

Stuart rubbed his eyes and stood as Lee took a seat behind a makeshift desk.

"Of course."

Lee laid out a map of the Shenandoah Valley and the

---

[23] Hand: in horse-talk, a hand is 4 inches.

Blue Ridge Mountain passes to the east. "When Joe Hooker finds out we're heading north into Pennsylvania, he'll react by heading north on the other side of the Blue Ridge Mountains. I'm sure they'll try to stay between us and the capital."

"Yes, I agree," Stuart said.

"After Chancellorsville, I don't think Hooker wants to fight. Longstreet and I want you to take three brigades of cavalry and head south behind them, then east, to outflank them. Once in position, you'll harass Hooker from the east. Do not engage him."

"You're sure you want to be without cavalry?" Stuart asked, his brow furrowed.

"No," Lee said. "But I think you can delay him enough that we'll meet on our terms, not his. We'll be okay 'til you return."

"Sooner or later, there will be a battle somewhere," Stuart surmised.

"I hope to meet him at Harrisburg where the mountains flatten into rolling hills," Lee said, pointing to Harrisburg, the capitol of Pennsylvania, which sat at crossroads in every direction. "If Hooker hurries out of Washington, it might be here," as Lee pointed to the smaller village of Gettysburg to the south. "Wherever we meet, I need to get there first and have time to set up defensive positions. If they rush north from Washington unprepared, we can attack them piecemeal one army at a time. After we crush Hooker again, I believe we can march on Washington and the Union will sue for peace."

Stuart nodded with a smile. "They must."

"Harass 'em, Jeb, that's all. Hooker will chase you a bit and buy us time."

"We'll leave at first light," Stuart replied and turned toward the tent flap.

"Ask the woman waiting outside to come in. It's the darndest thing. I've been told she's a surgeon with excellent skills," Lee said as he rolled the map.

"Yes," Stuart said, "She's one of the surgeons who

took care of us at Brandy Station. Dr. Romain, I think. She worked day and night after the battle. I thanked her for her service. Ewell wants you to give her a medal."

"That's what I heard," Lee responded as Stuart opened the tent flap and disappeared.

Rachel entered Lee's tent, stood in front of his desk and removed her sun hat. Lee's first serious look at her gave him pause, unprepared for her youth and attractiveness. She caught the glance but stood still, hands clasped together in front of her – quite unsoldierly.

"Dr. Romain, that's your name?" Lee asked.

"Yes, General. Quite right."

"I forgot you're a Brit. I heard of your father at Chancellorsville. He saw to General Jackson when he was seriously injured by our own men. Too late to help him, unfortunately."

"I was present as well and gave the anesthetic as Drs. McGuire and Guild removed his injured arm. Simon is my uncle and is back in Richmond recovering from typhoid."

"I hope he does well. Anyway, you and your uncle have stirred up a hornet's nest. A few of our surgeons want you gone, and now. You've angered them and they've threatened to leave. I've told them they'd be considered as deserters and arrested."

"If so, why haven't you asked us to leave?" Rachel said.

"Because the troops and my generals appreciate your efforts and do not want you gone. General Ewell even demanded I give you a medal. It presents a difficult situation for me." Lee's shoulders sagged, "As if that was my only burden."

"I'm sorry if we're a burden and I don't need or require a medal," Rachel said.

"How'd you two come to work for the Confederacy?"

"My uncle and I are studying the causes of infection after serious injuries sustained on the battlefield. We do not believe the current thinking that miasma is the culprit. We presented our theories to the Union but they wanted no part of us."

"Miasma? Explain that?" Lee asked, rubbing his chin.

"I'll tell you what others think. Miasma is contaminated or bad air. The miasma spreads and almost always leads to death."

"What is the cause then, if not bad air?" Lee asked.

"There's the rub, General. We're not sure," Rachel answered excitedly, her eyes glinting. "So far our studies have suggested that hand and instrument washing, along with isolation of one patient's wounds from others improves the odds of survival. We keep our amputees separate from the other surgeons."

"What have you found so far?"

"We've not had enough patients to be sure but my team's infection rate with amputation is less than seven percent. The other surgeons, together, average around twenty-five percent. Our study requires two hundred patients. We've reached one-hundred thirty-seven. After we've reached two hundred, Simon and I will return to London to present our findings at the Royal College of Surgeons."

Lee erupted, slamming his hand on the desk, surprising Rachel and causing her to jump backward. "You took an oath for the Confederacy, did you not?"

"Yes."

"But you would leave just like that, when our men need you? "They trust you," Lee said. "And you're doing damn good."

"Yes. We ... I believe we are doing good," Rachel said, realizing she needed to backtrack. "You've allowed us to do our research so I will help you how I can and won't leave you understaffed."

Lee said. "Good. I don't need a surprise exit of surgeons when I have no replacements. You need to promise me you'll stay until the battles are done through the fall.

Even if you reach two hundred before that," Lee said.

"My uncle needs to return to England to recuperate as soon as possible," Rachel insisted.

"You want to finish your research or not?" Lee demanded.

Rachel had no answer.

"Good. Dr. Romain, you're excused. Best be prepared, a huge battle is on the horizon."

With that, Lee turned his attention to papers on his desk. Rachel, realizing she'd been manipulated, said nothing else and left the tent.[24]

Rachel and Bessy arrived outside Gettysburg at the end of June and found Lafayette Guild two miles west on the Chambersburg Turnpike. Guild had taken over a large house and converted it into a general hospital. Rachel, Guild and seven other surgeons set up shop and awaited the battle.

---

[24] *That Lee believed, erroneously, that the apprehensive General Joe Hooker would still command the Union army only increased Lee's belief he would win again.*

When Union intelligence learned that Lee was heading north into Pennsylvania with seventy thousand men, Lincoln prodded Hooker to follow.

Lee didn't know that Lincoln would replace Hooker with George Meade, a Major General who believed the Battle of Chancellorsville could have been won if Hooker hadn't ordered a retreat. Meade took command of the Army of the Potomac as they headed north only three days before the Battle of Gettysburg would begin.

Lee had already made a fatal error by sending Jeb Stuart and his cavalry around and behind the Union army. By so doing, Lee lost his ability to scout the positions and strengths of the Union army. Lee arrived outside Gettysburg but didn't know Meade and ninety thousand troops of the Union Army of the Potomac were moving north, east of the Blue Ridge Mountains, only a day behind.

Lee's plan to arrive in Harrisburg first to establish defensive positions on higher ground never happened. He would need to fight in Gettysburg against a larger army and a general, George Meade, who would have the courage to stand and fight.

"Where's Heath and Clerk?" Rachel asked. "I'm starting to miss those two, although we agree on little."

"Funny, they asked about you as well and hope Simon is improving," Guild said. "Strange bedfellows we are. Anyway, they're a mile east of here, closer to the town."

"That could be dangerous," Rachel said.

"Yes, they know," Guild said. "Anyway, we need to get unpacked before..."

The unspoken hung in the air. They all knew that a devastating battle was inevitable.

Guild sat with Rachel that night for dinner on an operating table covered with a clean shroud instead of a tablecloth.

"This battle might decide the war," Guild said. "The casualties may be greater than anything we've seen yet."

"Then we have a huge problem, as I've checked our stores," Rachel said, softly shaking her head with concern. "We have far less chloroform than we did in Chancellorsville. You know we can't use ether at night with only candle power."

"We'll need to use ether during the day and limit chloroform usage to the night," Guild replied.

Rachel looked down at her plate; neither she nor Guild had much appetite. "If this battle is as bad as you think," she said, "we'll run out of both."

"All we can do now is hope that we rout the Yankees on the first day."

"I hate basing our ability to help injured men on hope," Rachel said. "It would be barbaric to run out of anesthetic. A return to the dark ages."

Guild could only nod.

Rachel did not hear cannon fire until 11 a.m. and the first ambulances didn't arrive until noon.[25] By then, the

---

[25] *Background – Battle of Gettysburg – Day 1* - July 1st 1863

surgeons, assistants, and anesthetists knew what was coming and what to do. She, Guild and the other surgeons, seasoned from prior battles, worked through the day, evening and into the wee hours of the morning.

At 3 a.m., Rachel, Bessy and Guild headed to their tents to gather what sleep they might.

"We've used half the ether and most of the chloroform," Rachel said to Guild. "If this goes on past

---

Believing Gettysburg to be unoccupied and guarded only by local militia, Confederate General Henry Heth sent infantry troops into town looking for a quick and easy victory. (It is a myth that the soldiers were only looking for shoes. But with myths, some things always ring true, as many Confederate soldiers were barefoot.)

Surprise awaited Heth's men in the form of Brigadier General John Buford and his small troop of Union cavalry. Buford was scouting a day ahead of the Union army's main force. Buford was surprised to see none of Jeb Stuart's cavalry. Buford knew that Meade and the Army of the Potomac would arrive that evening, which meant that the big battle to come would take place around Gettysburg, not Harrisburg as Robert E. Lee had hoped.

Though Buford's horsemen were dismounted and outnumbered, they had the new Spencer repeating rifle, which held seven cartridges in the buttstock and could fire twenty rounds per minute. The Confederate infantry troops used the Enfield single-shot musket which could fire, at most, only three rounds per minute. Believing they were facing a much larger force due to the rapid rate of fire received, the Confederates didn't advance.

The Battle of Gettysburg began in earnest as numbers of Confederate troops arrived from the west and north under General Richard Ewell while advance forces of the Union infantry under General John Reynolds arrived from the south of the city. The day ended as superior numbers of Confederates overwhelmed the smaller, front guard of the Union Army, forcing them to retreat.

Wisely, Buford had already scouted the area around Gettysburg. He had his small Union cavalry force retreat to the high ground of Cemetery Hill and Cemetery Ridge, south of Gettysburg. At midnight, George Meade and the bulk of the Union Army arrived.

Meade now controlled the high ground from Cemetery Hill to Little Round Top hill to Round Top hill – a distance of over two miles. Buford's actions this day, allowing the Union to hold the high ground around Gettysburg, helped decide the fate of the battle to come.

tomorrow, we'll be forced to do surgery without relief."

Guild's face was grave. "I've pleaded with General Lee's staff to find ether or chloroform. I have no idea whether they'll be successful."

July 2nd 1963

By 4 a.m. the ambulances slowed to a trickle.[26] "We'll never be able to handle all these injuries," Rachel complained to Guild. "We've almost run out of anesthetic."

"I know. I fear tomorrow may be worse," Guild said. "We'll need to use opiates to dull the pain and work quickly. I see no other answer."

"It's barbaric, Lafayette," Rachel shouted, rarely using Guild's first name. "The thought sickens me. I never would have come here knowing we can't ease the men's pain."

Lafayette Guild bowed his head as he had no answer for Rachel's concerns.

When Guild retired, Rachel rounded on the amputees for that day as Bessy logged them in.

July 3rd 1863

Rachel, Guild, Heath, Clerk and the other Confederate surgeons toiled through the night and the following

---

[26] *Background – Battle of Gettysburg – Day 2*
The Union forces had the high ground and were concentrated. The Confederate army wrapped around them except for the east side of the hills. Led by General James Longstreet, the Confederates assaulted the left flank of the Union, thought to be the hardest to defend. The Union general, Winfield Hancock, used his concentrated soldiers wisely, moving them like chess pieces to where they were needed. Battles raged at infamous places such as Little Round Top, Devil's Den, Peach Orchard, Culp's Hill, and Cemetery Hill. The casualties mounted on both sides. By nightfall, the Confederates had made little gain. More importantly, the Union Army continued to hold the high ground.

morning as ambulance after ambulance arrived at their hospitals[27]. They had run out of anesthetics and then opiates to offer relief to the injured men - after surgery, in the throes of death, and the unseen men awaiting treatment. Unrelenting screaming echoed from each operating room and from the acres of lawn outside the hospital.

The sheer number of injured men overwhelmed the hospitals. Floors were caked in pools of unclotted blood making traction impossible. Rachel and every member of the staff, covered in blood from the neck down, had repeatedly slipped to the floor.

Sleep deprivation and dehydration took its toll of the

---

[27] *Background – Battle of Gettysburg – Day 3*
Jeb Stuart finally rejoined Lee's army. The battle resumed on all fronts, including cavalry battles on the periphery of the Union lines. Robert E. Lee believed the center of the Union line was weakest on Cemetery Ridge and wanted to launch a frontal assault. General James Longstreet, Lee's second-in-command, argued that a frontal attack would be foolhardy but deferred to Lee. Meanwhile, George Meade predicted Lee would attack the center and prepared his infantry and artillery for such an attack. Meade's correct anticipation of Lee's strategy would help determine the outcome of the battle.

Lee sent General George Pickett and multiple Confederate divisions, totaling twelve-thousand-five-hundred men, to directly confront the Union forces on Cemetery Ridge over a mile of open ground with no cover. Blistering artillery and rifle fire decimated the Confederates. More than half of them were killed, wounded or captured. Pickett's Charge, as it came to be known, doomed Lee's army.

After the failure to take Cemetery Ridge, Lee feared a Union counteroffensive. When Lee asked Pickett to rally his division for a defense, Pickett reportedly said, "I have no division."

When a Union counterattack didn't occur, Lee understood that another assault made no sense. His army was barely subsisting off the Pennsylvania countryside with no way of replenishing itself, while the Union had the resources and men to mount a sustained counteroffensive. Lee ordered a retreat to Virginia.

By the third day of battle, over fifty-thousand men on both sides were killed, injured, missing or captured.

surgeons, assistants and aides. With less than four hours of sleep in three days, Rachel pleaded with Guild to rotate staff into shifts, allowing breaks of three hours to gather fluids, nourishment and rest. Guild agreed.

July 4th 1863

Lee's retreat had begun. After three days of battle, a tacit ceasefire settled over Gettysburg as ambulances on both sides collected the wounded. Rachel saw a higher percentage of Union injured soldiers than ever before.

On the evening of July 4th, retreating Confederates lined the road west to Cashtown. Heath and Clerk arrived at Rachel and Guild's hospital at 10 p.m. on horseback. Cloaked in blood, gaunt and unshaven, they looked no different than anyone still upright.

"Our hospital has been taken over by the Union cavalry," Heath shouted, watching Rachel as she closed the wound on an leg amputation with four aides holding the screaming man down. "Our sentries and guards put up a fight and were killed."

"But you escaped?" Guild asked, walking into the room.

"When the Yankee officers entered the hospital and saw we were surgeons," Clerk said, "they allowed us to leave if we took nothing."

"We've hundreds of injured men to care for and more coming," Rachel said breathlessly.

"Let the Yankees take care of 'em. You're crazy if you stay," Heath said. "We were lucky, I s'pose. Some of these Yankees have lost kin and friends. No promises they won't shoot you out of spite, surgeon or not. It's time for you to pack your things and head west on the Cashtown Road with Lee's main force, then south to Virginia while it's still possible."

"Will you wait for me?" Guild asked. "My wife is in Richmond. I, for one, will not suffer in a Yankee camp." Guild rushed out of the room to gather his personal belongings.

"I'm staying," Rachel said. "I have to finish my research or what my uncle and I have done here means nothing."

"You're either brave or stupid or both," Clerk said.

"Go, before I say something you and I will regret," Rachel replied. "I've work to do, so go if you must."

Guild returned holding a satchel of his surgical tools and started yelling to his men. "The Yankees will be here any moment. We must leave. Pack quickly and only the essentials."

Clerk went to the front door of the hospital, looking out for the arrival of Union cavalry.

Heath approached Rachel, his head bowed. "I was all wrong about you. You held your own as well an any could. Good luck. If I get to Richmond, I'll stop in and see how Simon fares."

"Thank you," Rachel said. "I'd appreciate that."

Before long, the three surgeons and their staff had mounted horses to head west toward Cashtown with the retreating Confederate army. They abandoned their wagons, most of their equipment, their tents, and ambulances of unseen injured soldiers for as far as the eye could see.

By nine p.m., Rachel had no more ether, chloroform, bandages, opiates, or sutures.

"What's we gonna do?" Bessy asked. "The ambulances be lined up fer as long as the eye can see. The drivers done unhitched their horses and rode off."

"Start tearing sheets into strips," Rachel said with tears in her eyes.

A few soldiers, strong enough to walk came to the door. All Rachel could do was offer comfort, salt water washes, and wrap strips of sheets over the open wounds.

At 3 a.m., absent even clean sheets, Rachel shut the door to the converted hospital. She and Bessy, caked in blood, sat against the wall away from the house's entryway.

"I'm too tired to look for clean clothing. We need some sleep," Rachel told Bessy. "Might as well be now until we get supplies somehow." In a side room near the front door, they found a small area on the floor without blood and sat. Leaning against the wall, both found sleep.

July 5th 1863
At 6 a.m., rifle shots shattered glass in the windows right and left of the hospital's front door. The shattered glass woke Bessy and she ran to the door, peeked out, then shut the door. Another bullet slammed through the door at chest level, missing her but showering her with wood fragments. Bessy ducked to the floor between the door and shattered window. Rachel, now awake, crawled to join Bessy.

"Lord help me, Miss Rachel, there be men on horses with guns and they be shootin' at us," Bessy shouted.

"Get me a large piece of any dirty white sheet," Rachel cried.

Bessy crawled into an operating room and returned with half a blood-soaked bed sheet which Rachel tore in half again.

Rachel crawled to the front door and slowly opened it a few inches, only to have a bullet enter the door a half inch above her hand. Undaunted, Rachel, on her knees, extended her hand out the door, waving the half sheet. She continued waving the sheet until she heard footsteps on the porch.

A deep voice yelled, "Drop your weapons and exit with your hands held high."

"We've got no weapons," Rachel yelled back. "We're a hospital!"

"Drop your weapons and exit with your hands held high," the deep voice repeated.

Rachel stood, holding the quarter sheet out the door, and stepped out onto the porch and held up her other hand. Ten Union soldiers, some on horseback, but all holding rifles or handguns, spread out in front of the house. All had their weapons trained on Rachel. A lieutenant with a flat hat stood five feet away, a pistol aimed at her head. He saw that Rachel was covered in blood and asked, "Are you injured?"

"No, I'm not. Put down those bloody guns," Rachel screamed. "I'm a surgeon. We have no arms. There are sick men inside as well as in those tents and ambulances around the house. They pose no threat."

"Stand away," the lieutenant said, "so we may check the house."

Rachel stepped to the side and the officer waved his men in, rifles and handguns held up and ready.

The lieutenant kept his pistol aimed at Rachel until one of the soldiers exited the house. "One dead and a few wounded men on tables, blood in pools on all the floors and walls and surgical instruments in each room. Most of the men are in pain. One of ours from Buford's brigade with a leg wound. He says the lady doctor's not a threat. He needs a surgeon bad. A black woman, also covered in blood and uninjured, says she works with the doctor."

The lieutenant said, "Ma'am, you'll have to come with us and explain it all to my captain."

"I'm not going anywhere, dammit," Rachel shouted. "Did you not hear me? There are countless wounded men, Union and Confederate, inside, in those tents, on the ground, and abandoned in the horseless wagons on the road. I need chloroform or ether, sutures and opiates. I have work to do."

"I don't know about that," the lieutenant said, "Think you oughta come with me."

"Damn you! Are you not hearing? Listen to me, I'm not leaving. If you've got any laudanum or morphine on you or your men, I need it. Your captain can bloody well come here and see what I have to treat."

"I'm only following orders, Ma'am," the lieutenant said. "I'll send one of my men to see what the Captain says."

"Thank you," Rachel said, lowering her voice. "Whilst we wait for your captain, might your men take the dead soldier and lay him out back and bring in another from the wagons?"

The lieutenant nodded and called over some men.

Twenty minutes later, another Union officer appeared in a plumed hat and a saber at his side. He found Rachel, still bathed in blood, attending a new man brought in with his leg shattered below the knee. Rachel had applied a tourniquet and given him some laudanum sourced from one of the Union soldiers.

"Ma'am, I'm Captain Morris Muscatel of Colonel Gregg's division. I've talked with my First Lieutenant who told me you weren't going to move until you took care of the injured men. That correct?"

"Damn right," Rachel said. "I'm Dr. Romain, a surgeon, and we need provisions and medical help."

"What do you need?" Muscatel asked.

"Chloroform or ether, sutures, bandages, nurses, aides and five or six surgeons," Rachel said, then added, "who know the hell what to do. There are hundreds of men, Confederate and Union, around this hospital on the ground, in tents and wagons. I need provisions and help. The equipment is here."

"Where are the rest of the Confederate surgeons, may I ask?"

"They fled when they heard you were near," Rachel said.

"You didn't," Muscatel asked. "Why?"

Rachel put her hands on her hips. "Injured men need care. I'm a British surgeon doing research on wound infection. I'm not a Confederate and I believe slavery is an abomination. But we're wasting time with these questions. I need provisions and help. If you or your men have any morphine or laudanum on you, I can start to work."

Muscatel became quiet, then turned to the

Lieutenant whom Rachel had met on the porch earlier, and barked orders, “Lieutenant, the medical supply depot is northeast of Gettysburg off the York Pike road. Take three men and bring back as much chloroform, bandages and sutures as they can spare. It’s no more than four miles there and back. I expect you back here within the hour.”

“Yes, sir,” the lieutenant replied. He tapped three men on the shoulder and they ran out the door to their horses.

Muscatel then turned to a sergeant. “William, take two men and a wagon and see if you can find Major John McNulty, the surgeon in charge of XII Corps. I have no idea where he might be now, but he was behind Culp’s Hill last night. Someone will know. Tell him we need surgeons and assistants here now. As many as he can spare.”

Ninety minutes later, Rachel, in clean clothing, had chloroform, sutures, bandages, and, most unexpectedly, a Union nurse named Catherine Canetti. Canetti, a Chicagoan attached to the 82nd Illinois Infantry, had been at the medical supply depot when she heard about the Confederate surgeon who needed assistance. She requisitioned a horse and rode back with Muscatel’s men.

Catherine, who liked to be called ‘Cat,’ was a dark-haired, 4-foot, 11-inch, ball-of-fire daughter of Brazilian immigrants and an abolitionist to boot. She and Rachel became instant friends.

Without hesitation, Rachel, Cat and Bessy went to work treating injured soldiers, Union and Confederate. Two hours later, a wagon with four surgeons, assistants and men arrived. While Rachel continued to operate, she had Cat start triaging injured men. Twenty hours of nonstop work later, Rachel told Captain Muscatel that she was hearing voices.

“Cat, Bessy and I need sleep,” she said, “before we make some terrible errors.”

Muscatel said, “Of course. I’ll be leaving tonight to rejoin my brigade. I’ve sent a man back to the medical supply depot to wire Washington that we need more supplies and surgeons. The Confederates have left five to six thousand injured men in the field and in their field hospitals.”

“Thank you for your support,” Rachel said.

“What you and the surgeons have accomplished in the past day is truly Herculean.” Muscatel then saluted Rachel and said, “It’s been my honor, Ma’am.”

Chapter Seventeen
An Undesirable
July 7th 1863

Rachel awoke at 6 a.m. after four hours of sleep. She shook Bessy and Cat awake and together they went down the stairs to find all the rooms occupied with surgeons, assistants, aides, and injured soldiers.

Rachel went outside to see if a kitchen had been established. On the porch, she met a major sitting on a chair with two sergeants beside him. The major stood as soon as he saw Rachel.

"Is there a kitchen set up yet?" Rachel asked.

"Yes, out back. I'm Major Richard Boxer and I assume you're Dr. Romain? We've been waiting for you."

"Yes, I'm Dr. Romain," Rachel said. "How can I help you?"

"I'm afraid I don't need your assistance," Boxer said, bowing his head. "We received a telegram at the medical depot. The Surgeon General, William Hammond, has commanded us to put you under arrest for entering the Confederate States illegally and providing support to the rebellion."

"That's madness," Rachel cried. "I'm here to help."

"So I understand," Boxer said, "and Captain Muscatel confirmed you've saved many lives and didn't shirk from your duties. But you broke the law by entering the Confederacy after you were warned that doing so was against the laws of the United States. You'll be able to plead your case to a judge in due time. You must come with me now."

Bessy and Cat came onto the porch, drawn out by the unfolding drama.

"Is this a joke?" Rachel screamed.

Boxer said, "No, it is not. Sergeant, please put handcuffs on Dr. Romain."

The sergeant removed oversized, wrought-iron handcuffs from his belt and approached Rachel, who stood paralyzed. Cat and Bessy, now fully understanding the situation, moved between Rachel and the approaching sergeant.

"Sergeant, you're making a mistake," Cat demanded. "We've work to do."

"Don't you dare touch this woman," Bessy yelled. "She be the most wonderful and hard-working white woman that ever be. She done nothing but good for me and my daughter and the soldiers, North and South, she and I takes cares of. This be wrong."

"Stand away," Boxer yelled, "or we'll arrest you too."

"Den you's gonna have to shoot me or takes me with Miss Rachel," Bessy cried. "She bought me fo' month ago and freed me the next day. She's promised to take me to Chicago City so as I can be with kin. If you leave me, I be a slave again or dead. Might as well shoot me now."

"Dr. Romain committed a crime," Boxer said sternly.

"Major," Cat said, "I'm a nurse attached to the Illinois 82nd. Dr. Romain is desperately needed here. Don't do anything until I can get one of the Union surgeons out here." Cat turned and ran back into the house.

"How can I lives in a place who hurt the peoples who has nuttin' but good in their heart?" Bessy cried as she backed next to Rachel, holding her arms around Rachel's waist. "She come here only to find out why mens die when they need surgery. She done that to help everyone. This be wrong. There be evil people all 'round here. Miss Rachel not one of 'em. She not have a bad bone in her body. Please. You go on your way now, hear."

Rachel kissed the back of Bessy's head and said, "Thank you."

"I'm sorry," Boxer said, "I can't do that. I've been given orders."

"Den y'all say y'all can't find her," Bessy said. "We haven't finished our work."

"Sergeants, remove this woman and put handcuffs

on Dr. Romain," Boxer said.

"Bessy," Rachel said, "You and Cat keep the log books going on the men we've operated on and the others. We can't lose months of research. You know what to do now."

"Yous taught me and Flora everything. I'll do it, Miss Rachel. I swears," Bessy said tearfully.

As the men grabbed Bessy by each arm, Cat returned with two surgeons and two assistants.

"Tell the major he's making a mistake," Cat said

Both surgeons said, "She's needed here, sir," in unison.

Boxer yelled at his sergeants, "Stop."

The men stood back but held onto Bessy. They looked to Boxer for orders.

"Dr. Romain," Boxer asked, "how long do you need to finish your research?"

"Seven more days on the men whom I and the other surgeons treated today. We'll know if the wounds are healing or not."

Boxer said, "If you give me your word of honor that you will not leave or try to escape, I'll return in a week to arrest you."

"I won't leave," Rachel said. "You have my word."

"Sergeant, let the woman go," Boxer said.

"Major, she's a damn Reb. She'll run," the sergeant with cuffs in hand said after releasing Bessy.

"She won't," Cat demanded. "I'd stake my life on it. Dr. Romain is dedicated to her research."

"I don't think she'll run, Sergeant," Boxer said. "She's given her word."

"I'll be here on this porch in a week. I promise," Rachel said.

Boxer tipped his hat, then he and his two sergeants headed off the porch toward their horses.

Bessy yelled at them as Boxer tipped his hat toward Rachel and Cat. "I be just as mad if y'all come back in a week, or a month or a year. Y'all hear me. Dis ain't right, no way, no how."

Rachel gave both Cat and Bessy a hug and a thank you, then headed around the house to find the kitchen.

Throughout the week, Rachel, Cat, Bessy and the other Union surgeons treated over six hundred men, a quarter of them Confederates. Cat triaged injured soldiers, Rachel taught surgical techniques to the less trained staff, and Bessy helped assistants with bandaging and holding the chloroform masks. At night, the three women would round on the men in the tents and on the ground and provide comfort and opiates when needed.

Rachel and Simon now had two-hundred-twenty-seven amputations where hypochlorite scrubbing and isolation has been used with a minimum of seven days of follow up. The other surgeons, Confederate and Union, had seven-hundred-twelve patients followed for at least a week.

Her research done, Rachel told Cat and Bessy, "Whatever happens to me, I've done the work I set out to do. I couldn't have done it without you."

The night before Major Boxer was expected to return to arrest Rachel, she and Cat sat after a midnight supper to talk. The subject came to love.

Rachel said, laughing, "I think I was in love with a patient during the battle in Chancellorsville."

"I don't believe you," Cat said. "You fell for a damn grayback?"

Rachel laughed again. "No. It was a captured Union officer who had been shot in the hand. I saw him twice but I just knew."

"He's in a prison camp now." Cat said.

"No. Before I had a chance to tell him how I felt, they told me he was swapped for a rebel officer. I have no idea if it's true, where he might be now or if he's alive. I expect that I'll never see him again."

"Strange, this war. Brother against brother," Cat said. "My family left Brazil in 1852 because they couldn't stomach slavery."[28]

"In any event, I've got to get packed in case that Major shows up to arrest me," Rachel said.

"I pray that he's forgotten about you," Cat said.

The next morning, July 18th, Major Boxer returned with the same two sergeants. Rachel and Bessy had already packed their belongings and surgical instruments. Cat, the surgical staff and the assistants knew what might happen and privately, to a man, they had hoped Boxer wouldn't return.

Again, Bessy stood between the sergeants and Rachel. "Dis be wrong, y'all hear me."

"Bessy," Rachel said, "Let it be. I gave my word so we could finish our research. Let it be."

"I wanna go with y'all," Bessy said as tears streamed down her face. "I gots no wheres to go."

"I'm sorry," Boxer said. "You've not broken any

---

[28] *Slavery ended in Brazil in 1888. Brazil was the last country in the Americas to allow slavery.*

President Lincoln was livid at General George Meade for not pursuing Lee after Gettysburg. In fact, Lincoln wrote a letter expressing his disappointment, but did not post it. That didn't stop the army chief of staff, General George Halleck, from letting Meade know how angry Lincoln had been. Lincoln had been angry at all of the generals of the Army of the Potomac up to that time for their timidity after battles, even if victorious.

Lee would not be able to cross the flooded Potomac River back into Virginia for another eight days. He had a severely depleted army, both in terms of men and supplies. The Union had reserves of men and equipment, but Meade hesitated, claiming he feared another attack. When the Union generals realized Lee had retreated, Meade thought his men were too exhausted to follow. Other than some minor cavalry skirmishes that week, the Battle of Gettysburg was over.

Some historians believe the war might have ended in 1863 if Meade had pushed his men to go after Lee, as Ulysses S. Grant would the following year after taking command of the Army of the Potomac.

laws."

Cat came onto the porch, instantly understanding that what she feared had come to pass.

One sergeant held up the wrought-iron handcuffs. When the other sergeant grabbed Rachel by the wrist, Bessy slapped him softly across the face. "Der, I's done hit a soldier. Y'all gotta arrest me too. I can't leave Miss Rachel."

Bessy held out her arms. "Put dos things on my hands. Miss Rachel a surgeon with magic hands. Y'all can't put no nothing on her hands."

"She's right," Cat said. "Dr. Romain isn't going to run. You can't put manacles on her."

Boxer shook his head. "God, I hate this. Okay, you two come with us peacefully without the handcuffs. The Union will provide you an attorney when it's time to make a plea to the court."

With tears streaming down her cheeks, Cat hugged Rachel and Bessy good-bye.

Rachel drew Cat aside and said, "After this debacle ends, Bessy and her daughter will try to find family in Chicago. Perhaps when you head home you might see that she's taken care of."

"Of course," Cat said. "I'll give her my family's address. As for you, I hope we meet again, as well."

As Cat scribbled an address for Bessy, Rachel thanked Boxer for letting her finish her research. Then she and Bessy followed Boxer and two guards out to the road.

By this time, Cat, the other surgeons and assistants had lined the porch, stairs and down the path. They stood in line, wishing Rachel and Bessy well.

Standing in a line further down the walkway to the road, a handful of injured Union men able to stand, stood shoulder to shoulder, heads bowed, as Rachel walked past. Each man said, "Thank you." The ones able to shake, shook Rachel's hands. Some of the Union soldiers whispered to Boxer as he passed, "Shame on you."

Rachel and Bessy were loaded onto the back of an open wagon and sat. When Rachel looked back, the injured men, as best possible, stood at attention and saluted.

Having no place to keep female prisoners, the army housed Rachel and Bessy in a tent near the medical depot. Two days later, both women were placed in a carriage with two sentries as guards.

The following day, Rachel and Bessy arrived in Washington, D.C. and transferred into the hands of Union jailers at the Capitol Prison, a three-story brick building which held Confederate spies and political prisoners. The jailers escorted the two women into the same cell. With non-existent ventilation, the prison air was rank with sweat, urine, and feces.

That night, a guard came to the cell after Rachel and Bessy had fallen asleep. He banged hard on the metal bars, awakening the women with a jolt.

The guard, smiling to have frightened them, said nastily, "There's a lawyer here to see you."

Rachel rubbed her eyes and sat up. "I didn't know I had a lawyer. Major Boxer told me one would be given to me tomorrow before we make a plea to the court."

"Dunno 'bout that, but he's here," the guard said.

Ten minutes later, Rachel and Bessy sat in a small, windowless room at the end of the cell block. In walked a well-dressed man, tall, brown hair parted in the middle, and steely brown eyes.

"Dr. Romain. Miss Bessy, I'm Robert Decker, an attorney. I've been sent to represent you by a close personal friend of yours."

"I know no one in the North who could be my friend except a nurse from Illinois named Catherine Canetti," Rachel said, confused. "Is this a trick? How much do your services cost?"

"It's not from an Illinois nurse. All fees for your

defense will be paid for by this friend," Decker said. "Every penny, or in your case, every farthing."

"Please tell me then who is my savior?" Rachel asked.

"I'm sworn to secrecy," Decker said. "This friend knows of your arrest and sent a telegram to Boston asking me to come to Washington to represent you. I'll be with you tomorrow but we need to spend an hour, first thing in the morning, so I can help you make a proper plea."

"I'm confused, the American court system is so different than that at home. You'll represent Bessy as well?"

"Of course. I expect her case to be dismissed tomorrow."

"I wants to stay with Miss Rachel," Bessy said. "If they lets me go, I be lost. She needs me too."

"Hopefully, that can be arranged," Decker said. "Either way, I'll make sure you're safe."

Decker left the room and the guard escorted Rachel and Bessy back to their cell.

"Who could it be that sent Mr. Decker?" Rachel mused.

"Don't knows," Bessy said. "Maybe Doctor Guild felt guilty leavin' us like that. Maybe that horrible Doctor Heath got some morals we didn't see. I dunno."

"Could be any of those injured men we treated or the surgeons or assistants who knew we were in the right. I can't think of anyone else who would even know I've been arrested other than Cat."

"S'pose it could be any of those. But I thanks the Lord fo' it."

"I have some hope now," Rachel said. "We can't go to jail. We need to get back to Uncle Simon and Flora."

"That fo' sure," Bessy said. "I hopes he and Flora be okay."

Early the next morning, Cat Canetti came to the jail with a basket of food for Rachel and Bessy. She wasn't allowed to see the prisoners, but wrote a note saying she'd be back every morning with food for them.

That morning, Decker met with Rachel and Bessy to learn of more of the charges against them. Later that day, Decker, Rachel and Bessy stood in front of a federal judge in the District of Columbia, The Honorable David Hartmon.

"If it pleases your Honor, I am Robert Decker, an attorney from the Commonwealth of Massachusetts who is representing Dr. Rachel Romain and Miss Bessy, a former slave who refuses to use her owner's surname."

"Thank you, Mr. Decker," Hartmon said, turning to Rachel. "Dr. Romain, I am here to read the charges against you as handed to me by the Attorney General of the United States, Mr. Edward Bates, who is represented by Mr. Theodore Burns here today."

Hartmon paused to make sure he had Rachel's attention. "Dr. Romain, you are charged with felonious entry into the United States after being warned not to enter. How do you plead?"

"Not guilty."

Hartmon continued, "Dr. Romain, you are charged with providing support for the rebellion against the United States after being warned not to do so. How do you plead?"

"Not guilty," Rachel said loud and clear.

"I assume you would prefer a trial by jury, Dr. Romain?" Hartman asked.

"My attorney, Mr. Decker," Rachel answered, "has suggested that I wave my right to a jury trial."

"Why is that? It is your right in the United States to be judged by your peers."

"My research is technical," Rachel said. "Much of the testimony in my defense might alarm or be misunderstood by some jurors, who are not my peers. You, Judge, are a man of letters and papers. I trust you will render a fair decision. I would appreciate a speedy trial date."

Hartmon smiled. “Dr. Romain, flattery will get you nowhere in this courtroom. But I can’t disagree with Mr. Decker’s logic. Miss Bessy, you are charged with slapping an officer of the United States Army. How do you plead?”

“I ain’t guilty of nutting but if’n I plead guilty, do I get to stay with Miss Rachel?” Bessy asked. “I knows I free now but I’s been a slave my whole life ‘til Miss Rachel buy me and my daughter, then free us the next day. I never been alone and got nowheres to go ‘cept staying with Miss Rachel. She be the only one who watch out fer me and I feels safe with her.”

Hartmon pondered the predicament then said, “I was going to dismiss all charges when I read the report, but then you wouldn’t be able to stay with Dr. Romain. I understand your devotion to each other, so I’ll accept your not-guilty charge for now. At Doctor Romain’s trial, I will dismiss the charges against you. If Dr. Romain is found guilty then you won’t be able to stay with her.”

“I still wants to be with her until she ready to go home across the sea,” Bessy said.

Hartmon nodded. “Of course.”

“Thank you, your Honor,” Decker said. “I’ve already told Miss Bessy I’ll see that she’s safe.”

Hartmon set a trial date for Monday, the 1st of August, seven days hence, but denied bail. In the meantime, Rachel and Bessy remained in jail but talked to Mr. Decker on a daily basis.

As promised, Cat brought a basket of food every morning for the five days. On the morning of July 30th a note in the basket said she’d be heading west with XI Corps and the Illinois 82nd Infantry into Tennessee that afternoon. She prayed that the trial would be decided in Rachel and Bessy’s favor.

July 31st 1863

On the day before the trial, Decker sat with Rachel and Bessy in the same windowless room down the hall from their jail cell.

Decker said, "I've talked to Mr. Burns about dropping the charges, but they wish to make a point of it by going to trial. The Attorney General doesn't believe we have a defense."

"If we lose, how much time might I spend in jail?" Rachel asked.

"That's up to the judge. You're not a spy. My guess is no more than a year, but it could be as long as ten years."

"Ten year!" Bessy cried. "I thinked that judge be nice but I give him a piece o' mind if he do anything like that."

Decker laughed. "Bessy, you may find yourself in jail with Dr. Romain after all. I've seen the letter and the response from Doctors Letterman and Hammond. They did warn you not to come and that helping the South meant you were providing aid to them."

"I came for a higher purpose," Rachel said. "I believed this research too important not to be done. I would have come to the North but they prevented me. If I'm guilty of saving human lives, then I can live with that. I know English history. The American Revolution was against the laws of Britain. But the colonists appealed to a higher law and fought for their freedom. It was too important for them not to."

"May I use that statement about saving lives in my closing to the judge?" Decker asked.

"You may," Rachel said. "Who will be at the trial? I have no one who will support me other than you."

"I've been busy rounding up men you've helped," Decker said. "You have more support than you know. Wait 'til tomorrow."

August 1st 1863

The courtroom of David Hartmon was packed with wounded veterans from the Battle of Gettysburg. Many were missing limbs while others wore head bandages, but all wore the uniform of the Union army. Rachel, Bessy and Decker sat at a table opposite Ted Burns, the Assistant Attorney General.

The bailiff stood at the back of the courtroom and announced, “All rise. The Federal District Court for the District of Columbia is now in session; the Honorable David Hartmon, presiding.”

Hartmon entered, climbed to his bench and said, “All be seated.”

Ted Burns presented the government’s case in less than ten minutes. He read a copy of the letter sent to Simon Romain from Drs. Letterman and Hammond then repeated the warnings given to Simon and Rachel:

> “The United States Army received your and your niece’s request to perform experiments on our troops. We have no time for such nonsense. In addition, as your experiment gives succor to the enemy, you will not be given permission to enter or provide aid to any of the illegal Confederate states.”

“Judge,” Burns continued, “This letter is signed by Dr. William Hammond, Surgeon General of the United States and Dr. Jonathon Letterman, Medical Director of the Army of the Potomac.”

Burns handed the letter to Hartmon, then continued. “Both Dr. Simon Romain and Dr. Rachel Romain entered the United States illegally by Dr. Rachel Romain’s own admission and, by Dr. Rachel Romain’s own admission, she and her uncle aided the war against the United States by providing surgical and medical services to the rebellious and illegal Confederate army.”

Burns hesitated for emphasis, then concluded, “Your Honor, the United States needs to prove nothing else to show the guilt of the Romains and we rest our case.”

Hartmon said, “Well, that was short. Thank you, Mr. Burns. Mr. Decker, your defense.”

Decker stood and said, “We’d like to call Dr. Rachel Romain to the stand.”

Rachel approached the witness stand and as she did all the injured veterans who could do so stood, often aided by the men next to them. Together, they saluted her.

“Impressive, Mr. Decker,” Hartmon said, smiling. “But this is a courtroom not a theater. All be seated.”

After being sworn in by the bailiff, Rachel took her seat and Decker approached. As Rachel scanned the courtroom, she spotted a tall man in a Union Army officer’s uniform standing by the exit. He wore a full-sized, military slouch-hat with gold embroidery near the back. When their eyes met, the soldier held up a gloved left hand, waved, then lowered his hand and walked out of the courtroom.

Rachel stared at the empty doorway, waiting for the officer to return. Was the little finger missing, she asked herself? Could it really have been Solomon Birch, the quartermaster officer who had returned to the Union in a prisoner swap? Had he come in her defense? But he left without a word. Who was it?

“Dr. Romain,” Decker said and repeated louder, “Dr. Romain.”

Rachel, coming out of her trance, looked at Decker.

“Dr. Romain, in your own words, tell the court why you entered the United States and worked for the Confederate Army.”

Rachel sat up and, in a clear voice, began her own defense. “My uncle and I, working as surgeons in London, took a sabbatical for six weeks to Europe in 1861. In Budapest, and quite by accident, I met an obstetrician named Ignaz Semmelweis and this is what he told me ...”

For the next two hours, Rachel explained Semmelweis’s research and findings, then her return to London and the resistance she faced from other surgeons when attempting to prove those findings.

"My uncle and I were frustrated because, if true, Semmelweis's findings could save thousands of people from infection of wounds and death."

"Why is it that no one believed you?" Decker asked.

Rachel responded, "Because believing so would change the time-honored belief that miasma or 'bad air' was the cause of infection. We didn't know why Semmelweis's techniques worked and neither did he. Absent an exact reason, doctors refused to believe its value."

Decker asked, "Why did you need to come to the United States to prove your hypothesis?"

"We needed large numbers of patients with similar wounds to collect the data. That had been pointed out to us by one of our biggest detractors, Sir Michael Diamond, the head of the board at our hospital, St. James Charity, in London. He said that for us to do our study, we would need France to invade England and hope we had enough war injuries at the same time to make our analysis valid."

"France did not invade England?" Decker asked.

"No, but a war began in the United States," Rachel said. "We first asked only the Northern states if we might do the study at no cost to them."

"What was their response?" Decker asked.

"Mr. Burns read their response. *We have no time for such nonsense*, they said."

"What did you think of that?"

"Quite rude. We wanted to reduce the mortality of injured soldiers on the battlefield. At worst, our results would be the same as the other Union surgeons. At best, the mortality rate would plummet, thereby saving countless lives."

"So, what next?" Decker asked.

"Only then did we write the same letter to the Southern States and they agreed to have us come. So we came. We found a blockade runner to sneak us in."

"You admit to that?" Decker asked.

"Yes."

"What did you find out in your study?"

"We controlled our surgeries and those of the other surgeons, Confederate and Union, to amputations only done within forty-eight hours of injury so the procedures, methods and materials would be comparable. Simon and I performed two-hundred-twenty-seven amputations of the leg and arm where hypochlorite scrubbing and isolation had been used with a minimum of seven days of follow up. The other surgeons had seven-hundred-twelve patients without the use of hypochlorite scrubbing or isolation. All the patients were followed for at least a week. Our infection rate was five point two percent. The other surgeons had a twenty-three-point-three percent infection rate."

"Quite significant, I think?" Decker asked.

"Yes. It's not miasma. It's not the bad air. The cause of the infection is something localized to the surgeon's hands or instruments or the patient's skin, I believe."

"But you're not sure exactly?"

"Not yet, but if we keep looking, we'll find it," Rachel said. "We've never known where to look before."

"What would you do next?" Decker asked.

"Simon and I should return home and publish our study in a journal and present our findings to the Royal College of Surgeons. We would hope others would confirm our findings and then start looking for the reason why hypochlorite scrubbing saves lives."

"Dr. Romain, I believe that's all we need to discuss," Decker said.

Hartmon turned to Burns and asked, "Would you like to cross examine Dr. Romain?"

Burns stood and said, "No, Your Honor. The prosecution rests. I believe I can present a closing now."

"You may proceed," Hartmon said.

"Dr. Romain has proven our point. I don't care how important she feels her research was or how rude our Surgeon General might have been in a letter. The

Romains entered the United States illegally and then provided aid to the rebellion. It's as clear as crystal and she admits it. She's guilty as sin. Your honor has no choice but to find Dr. Romain guilty as charged on both counts.

With that, Burns took his seat, looking smug.

"Mr. Decker, your closing," Hartmon said.

"Yes, your Honor," Decker said. "I've been a lawyer for over twenty years now and have made countless closing statements. Some quite eloquent, I must say."

The courtroom laughed, as did Judge Hartmon, and even Ted Burns.

Decker continued, "Dr. Romain and I discussed her situation and here's what she told me. I wrote it down verbatim as soon as I left her presence." Decker paused and picked up a sheet of paper and read from it. "She said, 'I came for a higher purpose. I believed this research too important not to be done. If I'm guilty of saving human lives, then I can live with that. I know English history. The American Revolution was against the laws of England. But the colonists appealed to a higher law and fought for their freedom. It was too important for them not to.'"

Decker paused. "I could not have composed a better closing argument to find Dr. Romain innocent. The defense rests, you Honor."

Hartmon said, "Thank you both for your brevity. I'll retire to my chamber and give this some thought. I won't be long in making my decision." Hartmon stood, left the bench and entered his chamber.

"What now?" Rachel asked Decker.

"Hard to know. I assume he'll be back shortly, so we should stick around. You, however, are not free to leave the courtroom."

"Might someone from the crowd talk to me here?"

"Yes," Decker said.

Rachel stood and scanned the crowd, looking for the man who waved. She realized the mystery man could have been any one of the Union soldiers she'd treated those last days around Gettysburg, or even coming from a thankful family of someone injured. But she recognized no one in the courtroom. Rachel frowned, returned to her seat and leaned over to Bessy. "For a moment, I thought I figured out who had paid for Mr. Decker. It was that officer, Solomon Birch, at Chancellorsville."

Bessy nodded. "The one missing fingers."

Rachel said, "I saw some man waving and I thought it might be him. But he left without even a hello. So it's a mystery."

"You be dreamin', I s'pose, Miss Rachel," Bessy said. "Best not git y'all hopes up too much. I'd be worryin' right 'bout now whether you goin' to jail."

Twenty minutes later, the bailiff again called order in the court. "All rise."

Rachel whispered to Bessy, "I'm so nervous I could vomit."

"Everything gonna be all right," Bessy whispered back. "I just feels it."

Hartmon resumed his seat at the bench and said, "All seated. When everyone had taken their seat, he said, "Will the defendants please rise."

Rachel, Bessy and Decker stood. Rachel held onto Bessy's upper arm for support.

Hartmon began, "This was a difficult case for me to decide. Laws were broken but for reasons only a dedicated surgeon and scientist would know. Still laws were broken and we are a nation of laws. In the case of the United States of America versus Dr. Rachel Romain, I find Dr. Romain guilty on the charge of entering the United States illegally and guilty in aiding the States in rebellion."

"Dat ain't right," Bessy yelled.

"Shhh," Decker said. "You'll find yourself in jail."

Hartmon continued after glaring at Bessy. "Doctor Romain, I hereby sentence you to twelve days in jail, the amount of time you've already served."

"Dat's better, I guess," Bessy said.

Hartman again stared down Bessy who bowed her head in contrition.

Hartman continued, "Normally, Dr, Romain, in these situations as a foreign citizen who has broken a serious law, you would be extradited back to your own country as soon as your prison term has been completed. However, I assume you need to wait for your uncle to recuperate before that happens. Is that correct?"

"Yes, your Honor. I cannot leave without him."

"In that case, you are free to remain in the United States until your uncle is free to travel. When that occurs, I suggest you head back to England at the soonest possible time. If you delay your departure for any reason, I assure you the Department of Justice will force you to leave. Is that understood?"

"Yes, your Honor," Rachel said.

"As for you, Miss Bessy," Hartman said, "you've already spent too much time trying to protect Dr. Romain. I am dismissing the charges against you. You are also free to go." Hartmon banged his gavel, stood, and exited the court.

As soon as the door to Hartmon's private quarters closed, Ted Burns slammed his fist on his table and muttered, "Damn that judge."

Rachel turned to Decker, "What does that mean? I'm guilty but free to go?"

Decker smiled. "You broke the law and he had to find you guilty so the U.S. Attorney could go back to his boss and say he won the case. But he sentenced you to twelve days in jail, the time you've already spent in custody. So you're free to go."

"Amazing," Rachel said. "Then why did they arrest me in the first place?"

"Because you broke the law," Decker said. "I would, in the strongest terms, tell you to be careful and not break any more laws. The Attorney General will not be pleased about this result and the courts and a new judge might not be so lenient in the future if you break any of our laws in any way."

"I thank you," Rachel said. "I'm certain this wouldn't have turned out so well without you."

"You're welcome," Decker said. "I can see why my benefactor wanted me to defend you. It's my honor to have aided you."

"Now will you tell me who sent you?" Rachel asked.

"My instructions were quite clear," Decker said. "I am not to divulge the identity of my employer. I can tell you that my family and the family of your benefactor go back to before the American Revolution. So this was a bit of payback for years of mutual help."

"Will I ever learn who aided me?" Rachel asked.

"That's your benefactor's decision, not mine," Decker said with a shrug.

"Very well," Rachel said. "It's time that Bessy and I return to our relatives in Richmond."

"That's complicated. We're still at war and you must not try to return to Richmond without clear authorization," Decker said. "You, Bessy and I will need to go to the Department of War and make your plea to see if they can work out a way for you to have safe passage to Richmond and back with the promise that once you've retrieved your uncle, you'll leave the United States and return home to England immediately."

Rachel and Bessy, now free, checked into a hotel in Washington booked by Decker.

The next morning, a visit to the War Department revealed that all prisoner exchanges had ceased as of June that year. They didn't know when the exchanges would resume and until that time, there was no way to retrieve Simon and Flora from Richmond.

"What now?" Rachel asked.

"You wait," Decker said. "I'd recommend checking with the War Department every so often. Technically, your uncle and Bessy's daughter aren't prisoners of war but I know no other guaranteed means of safe passage during wartime. As you, Bessy and your uncle will no longer work for either side, I believe it will be easily agreed to. I'd wait for exchanges to resume."

"Where will you go now?" Rachel asked.

"Back to Boston and resume my practice. My train leaves this afternoon," Decker said. "Will you and Bessy stay in Washington?"

"Don't know. Bessy doesn't want to move to Chicago until Flora is freed."

"Dat's fo sure," Bessy said.

"You may want to rent a house somewhere nearby," Decker said. "The hotel wasn't too keen on having Bessy stay there."

"Dat's fo sure too," Bessy said. "I's not welcome."

At dinner that night with Bessy, Rachel fidgeted the entire meal.

"What's be wrong with you," Bessy asked. "You actin' likes you be sittin' on a sliver 'o wood."

"I'm worried about Simon. We don't know how he's doing. And Flora too," Rachel said.

"Nah, that be the same fo' a spell now," Bessy opined. "It's somethin' else."

"I thought I'd figured out who hired Mr. Decker, but if it was Solomon Birch, then why did he come only to leave without a word?"

"S'pose he had to be somewhere else," Bessy said. "Now that you been thinking on it, I remember befo' we put him to sleep he told me his mama gots ether for some surgery she had in Boston city. Dat's where Mr. Decker from. So, I'm thinkin' it might be him."

"Let's go to Boston then," Rachel said. "We've got time, and we can come back here in a week or two to see whether we can get back to Richmond."

"If Mr. Birch be in army uniform," Bessy said, "he ain't gonna be in Boston. They ain't fightin' in no Boston."

"Possibly, but I can't stand the thought of waiting around here doing nothing."

"Miss Rachel, you something. My whole life I didn't go nowheres but town and the plantation. Dat's it. Since I met y'all, I been goin' everywheres."

The next morning, Rachel and Bessy packed their luggage and went to the front desk to check out.

"Miss Romain," the clerk said, his eyes lighting up, "we received two letters for you this morning." The clerk turned and removed the posts from a room slot and handed it to Rachel.

The first envelope read only 'Dr. Rachel Romain.' Rachel opened the letter and read.

> *August 12. 1863*
> *Dear Dr. Romain,*
> *First of all, I am well and the wounds to my hand have healed nicely. I'm sorry I couldn't stay longer at your trial. My division was boarding a train on the way south as the trial commenced.*
> *A friend telegraphed me that you had been released. It is only fair that you were not sent to prison. A courier from our unit was heading to Washington last night and I gave him this letter to deliver to you.*
> *I will be back in Washington on September 1st on a two-week leave. Hopefully you will still be there as we've stories to share. Thank you again for the extraordinary care I received.*
> *Sincerely,*
> *Major Solomon Birch*
> *Quartermaster, First New York*
> *United States Army*

Rachel folded the letter and replaced it in the

envelope. She turned to Bessy with a huge smile. "It's from Solomon Birch. It was him. He'll be back in Washington in two weeks' time and is anxious to see me. We don't need to go to Boston."

Rachel then opened the second letter, which had her name and the Department of War on the outside.

August 14. 1863
Dr. Rachel Romain,
Please arrive at the Department of War office on Monday, August 17, 1863 at 9 a.m. We have important information about Dr. Simon Romain and his nurse."

Colonel Bruce Backer
Office of the Commission General of Prisoners

"What dat say?" Bessy asked.

It's from the War Department. They want me to be at their office on Monday. It's about Simon and Flora."

"Is dat good or bad?" Bessy asked with a worried expression "I pray dey be okay."

"Doesn't say, but let's hope it's good. We'll need to return to our room and see what tomorrow brings." Rachel informed the hotel clerk they'd be staying for a few more days.

At 9 a.m. on Monday morning, Rachel appeared at the War Department and asked to speak with Colonel Bruce Backer. An armed soldier escorted her up two flights of stairs and into the office of Colonel Backer, a portly, heavily bearded gentleman of about fifty dressed in a crisp Army officer's uniform. The armed soldier stood at attention outside the door.

'You're Dr. Rachel Romain?" Backer asked.

"Yes," Rachel replied.

"Have a seat." Backer said as Rachel took a seat

across from him. "I've been in contact with a General Kevin Beauregard," Backer said, "who holds the same position as mine only in the Confederate States. It's a most unusual situation. As a rule, neither side has kept doctors as prisoners. They were felt to be non-combatants. Anyway, Beauregard and the Confederates wish to swap a surgeon we captured after Gettysburg trying to escape."

"I'm not going back to serve in their army," Rachel said. "I've completed my research."

"So I understand," Backer said. "They wish to swap your uncle, Dr. Simon Romain and his servant, for Dr. John Heath, a surgeon from Alabama."

"I know Dr. Heath," Rachel said.

"Of course you do. You worked on their side against us," Backer said, shaking his head.

"It's not like that. I was doing research."

"So you say. I've spoken with Mr. Theodore Burns from our Department of Justice and he explained your situation. I might add he believes the judge was extremely lenient. Burns expected you to go to prison for a good deal of time. Anyway, we've agreed to swap Heath for your uncle and servant."

"That's wonderful," Rachel said.

"We've shipped Dr. Heath off last night on a Union Navy boat to Richmond under a flag of truce. Dr. Romain and his servant will be placed on the same boat and shipped back from Richmond to here. I expect he'll arrive by tomorrow morning at the Sixth Street Wharf."

"This is so unexpected. That's wonderful news," Rachel said.

"Perhaps, perhaps not," Backer said with a smirk. "By Mr. Burns' instructions, as undesirables to the United States, you and your uncle will be sent to Baltimore as soon as he arrives and held there. You both will be deported on the first ship that sails for any port in England. You and your uncle will never be allowed to return to the United States.'"

"Damn it all. My uncle and I are not undesirables," Rachel seethed. "Besides, my uncle is recuperating from typhoid. He's in no shape to travel across the ocean."

"You and your uncle," Backer said, with anger in his eyes, "were found guilty of entering the United States illegally and furthermore found guilty of aiding the rebellion. Your uncle has not faced a Union judge for the same crimes. By any definition I can think of, you and your uncle are both undesirables and you are lucky not to find yourselves in a Union prison. End of story. If your uncle is alive, then he's in good enough shape to get on the first ship to England. You must appear at the Sixth Street Wharf at 9 a.m. tomorrow. If you do not appear, you will be found and arrested for remaining in the United States illegally and your uncle will stand trial for the same crimes."

"What of our servants? They are freed slaves," Rachel asked, trying to maintain her composure.

"They've not been found guilty of a crime as far as I know," Backer said. "They're free to go wherever they damn well please. Take 'em to England as far as I'm concerned."

"But I have a meeting on September 1st," Rachel said. "I'll show you the letter. It's from a Union officer whose life I saved and ..."

Backer interrupted Rachel. "You're not listening, Dr. Romain. I said appear with your luggage at the Sixth Street Wharf tomorrow at 9 a.m. An army officer assigned to your uncle expects you there. The officer will transport both of you to Baltimore. Trust me that the Department of Justice will arrest and imprison you if you're not there. Your uncle will be shipped home with or without you."

Rachel, stunned, didn't know what to say. She sat mutely looking at Backer.

Backer broke the silence. "I'm busy and we've reached the end of our conversation. Nine a.m., Sixth Street wharf. I'll have you escorted out."

Back at the hotel room with Bessy, Rachel strode back and forth the length of the bedroom screaming over and over, "The sons of bitches. I am so damn furious!"

"I thinks you gotta calm down, Miss Rachel" Bessy pleaded. "Ders a whole lot of good in what's happened. "Y'all gots to look on the bright side. Count 'em. Mr. Simon probably be better, Flora be coming back, we's not slaves no mo', y'all research got done, y'all didn't go to jail, and y'all get to go home. Sounds good to me."

"I suppose," Rachel said. "I lost one man I was going to marry in a freak accident. Solomon is the first man since my Andrew died that made me even think I'd find someone else. Maybe I was being naïve."

"I don't know what naïve means."

"Foolish."

"I s'pose," Bessy said, "you just needs to leave a message at the hotel desk fo' Mr. Birch how to reach y'all and tell dat Mr. Birch what happened. If he be the right man for you, he'll lets you know, somehow."

Rachel stopped pacing and said, "I don't even know if he only wanted to say thanks or if he wants more. All I wanted was see him once more."

"What be done is done. Not like you to complain when ders nuttin' to do 'bout it. I seen you with injured soldiers comin' in each door and window at the same time and you be calm as can be. Dis ain't nuttin' and yous all up and down."

"I'm sorry," Rachel said. "You're right."

Let's get y'all packed fo' tomorrow. Gotta do that anyways. Den you gots to take me to the train station and help buy me and Flora a ticket to Chicago town."

Bessy then held up a money order made out to her. "I gots a twenty dollar cash in my bag and alls I need to do is shows dis piece o' paper in a Chicago Post Office[29]

---

[29] The U.S. postal money order system originated in the 1860s to provide a safer way to send money through the mail, particularly for Civil War soldiers.

and dey give me and Flora all the moneys we been paid for free?"

Rachel nodded.

"I hope," Bessy said, "that alls the white people in Chicago town be as nice as you."

"Some will be, some will not," Rachel said. "You'll need to learn from your family whom you can trust. Keep your money in a bank, a big bank. It will be difficult for you and Flora in the beginning, but because you both can read and write, you should be able to manage. You might even be able to find a job in a hospital with your experience. Cat comes from Chicago and may be able to help you after the war."

"I hope so, Miss Rachel. I wish y'all could come with us."

Rachel laughed at the comment. "I'm not welcome in this country. You and Flora would have to come to England. But I needed family to make my life complete. I think you and Flora will need that too and that's in Chicago."

They hugged, tearfully, for a long time.

Rachel and Bessy arrived at the Sixth Street Wharf at ten to nine in the morning, where they headed to the only ship docked. Rachel saw a single armed sailor standing guard at the roped-off gangplank.

Rachel called to the guard. "Ahoy. My name is Rachel Romain and I am expected here at 9 a.m. to meet a naval officer."

"Most everyone is off the ship, Ma'am," the sailor said.

"My uncle is supposed to be on board," Rachel said. "He's recovering from typhoid."

"I just got here and I can't leave my post, Ma'am. You'll need to wait for someone to come up on deck who can see if there are still passengers below."

Bessy decided to take matters into her own hands, screaming, "Flora, Flora. You come on out now!"

A second later, they heard: "Mama, I be coming," ring from somewhere on the ship followed by Flora opening a door and bursting onto the deck.

A tall, naval officer followed her, approaching the gangplank and yelling down, "Are you Dr. Romain's niece?"

"Yes. Where is my uncle?" Rachel asked.

"He's below deck in a bunk," the officer said. "I'm afraid he's a bit too weak to climb the stairs. We'll need some sailors to carry him. Would you like to come up?"

"Absolutely," Rachel said as she ran up the gangplank past the guard.

No sooner was she on board that Flora hustled down the gangplank into her mother's arms.

Rachel followed the officer down a set of stairs and found Simon lying on his back in a low bunk. She gasped at the sight of him. He had not regained any of the weight he'd lost. Worse, his skin appeared grayish, semi-lucent, and taut. When he saw Rachel, he smiled painfully.

"I missed you," he said in a low monotone.

"Not as much as I missed you," Rachel replied, sinking to his bedside. "How do you feel?"

"Better than I did a week ago. Flora has taken good care of me. No more fevers or diarrhea."

"We're being deported from the United States. Did you know that?" Rachel asked.

"So they told me," Simon whispered. "We're to be put on a boat to Liverpool in Baltimore. Did you finish the study?"

"Yes. The data is solid. We'll discuss it when you're stronger."

Simon nodded, then closed his eyes.

Rachel turned to the officer, a naval lieutenant commander. "In my opinion as a physician, my uncle is in no shape to travel even to Baltimore, let alone endure an arduous sea journey."

"Ma'am, my commanding officer met with Colonel

Backer and I have my orders. If you and your uncle are not on the ship by tomorrow, I'm to have you both arrested and brought back to Washington so your uncle can stand trial."

"Is that some kind of a joke?" Rachel begged.

"You had a trial," the officer said, "According to Backer, your uncle has not. Can't promise he'd be as lucky as you with a different judge."

Rachel shook her head in despair. She had lost her last chance to stay in Washington and meet Solomon Birch.

Off the ship, as sailors loaded Simon into an ambulance, Rachel said her tearful good-byes to Bessy and Flora. Before long, she was waving at the cab that would take them to the west side of Washington to start the arduous train journey to Chicago. Rachel then joined Simon in the ambulance to be taken to the railroad station on the east side of Washington.

In Baltimore, sailors carried Simon's stretcher onto the *Golden Bear*, a three-masted British tea clipper, and then carried him down a flight of stairs into a small apartment. Having noticed that the ship was listing slightly, Rachel sought out the captain. The *Golden Bear*'s captain, Edward Atkins, didn't believe for one second that Rachel knew anything about ships.

"You're listing a point to the port," Rachel said. "You might want to rearrange your cargo," she said.

Atkins's eyes narrowed. "You must have heard that from one of my men. We're taking care of it," Atkins whined. "Besides, women cannot wander about this ship or help in any way. Lloyd's of London demand only experienced seamen under our flag."

"Ask me anything about this or any other ship," Rachel said. "Or any port from Cape Town to Osaka."

Thirty minutes of discussion later, Atkins apologized. Rachel changed into her linen naval togs and bare feet for the rest of the voyage.

Each day, Simon improved and was able to walk the deck by the time the *Golden Bear* docked in Liverpool early on the morning of August 20th 1863. Once docked, Rachel sent a telegram to Cynthia that they would be in London that evening.

Simon said, "You must let me walk off the train myself. Cynthia will take one look at me and start crying or yelling or both."

They arrived in London six hours later. Cynthia stood on the platform, waiting. Seeing Rachel aid Simon off the train onto the platform, Cynthia ran to greet them. She gave Simon a hug then held him at arm's length and said, "Look at me. This is not who I said good-bye to last March."

"I'm here," Simon said, "and getting better each day. I'm recovering from typhoid."

"As I live and breathe, Simon Romain, you look like death warmed over," Cynthia barked. "You both have hours of explaining to me how this could have happened."

"We did finish our research," Rachel said.

"You left Simon alone to do research?" Cynthia said, knowing the answer.

"For a short time," Rachel lied.

Cynthia swiveled to confront Rachel. "At what cost? I know typhoid as well as anyone. You both promised to stay together. My husband almost died." Cynthia's glare told Rachel all she needed to know and the research wasn't mentioned again for three weeks.

Chapter Eighteen
Royal College

Rachel returned to work at St. James Charity within a few days of arriving back in London.

Meanwhile, at home, Cynthia and Sharron devoted themselves to fussing over Simon, preparing easily digestible foods to aid in his recuperation from typhoid: water and juices, porridge, boiled eggs and bland broths.

Every evening, Rachel and Simon would recount to Cynthia bits of their journey to the American South. When they arrived at the time after Chancellorsville when Simon became sick, Rachel's decision to continue the research and leave Simon with Flora did not sit well with Cynthia.

"Did you not consider staying with Simon, as you promised, rather than galivanting off?" Cynthia asked. "I sent him with you to make sure you'd be looked after. I assumed you'd do the same for your uncle!"

"He was on the mend," Rachel said sheepishly. "He encouraged me to go."

"I did," Simon said. "I demanded that she go."

"Damn you both and damn the research," Cynthia said, out of character. "What were you thinking? You stay together at all costs."

Rachel knew not to argue and could only say, "I'm sorry, Mum."

Simon gained strength and weight each day and within a month declared, "I'm ready to go back to work."

"Not on your life." Cynthia said. "You are not returning to work until you've regained every pound lost. You still have a ghostly look to you and you'd frighten the patients, doctors and nurses who know you. It scares me how badly this could have ended."

Rachel had misjudged how unhappy Cynthia would be about Simon's illness and stayed clear of her aunt as much as possible.

One evening after Simon had fallen asleep, Rachel and Cynthia found themselves sitting together in the parlor.

"Would you like me to leave?" Rachel said.

"No, of course not," Cynthia said.

"Will you ever forgive me?" Rachel asked.

"I already have. But I hope you've learned something."

Rachel waited, knowing Cynthia had more to say.

"When you are married," Cynthia said, "and if you have children of your own, you'll remember this episode and think, 'How could I have abandoned Simon?'"

"We did discuss it," Rachel said. "Simon implored me to go and finish the research."

"Let me ask you this. If Andrew had not died but had been seriously injured and needed round-the-clock care, would you have gone off to America, even if he said you should go?"

"No, I suppose not," Rachel said.

"Why did I demand that Simon go with you? For this very reason. We are family and protect loved ones at all costs."

Rachel nodded. "You're right. I'm sorry."

After a few seconds of silence, Cynthia said, "Now tell me about this Solomon Birch again. The man with eight and a half fingers."

Rachel smiled, understanding that Cynthia had said her piece.

A month later, Simon had regained all his weight and color and re-opened his office. Cynthia knew he still lacked stamina and insisted upon half-time work for the next month before returning to a full work week.

Together, Simon and Rachel started working on the data from America. Rachel had told her surgical colleagues about the results, but none showed interest in scrubbing their hands with hypochlorite solution. The nurses at the two Romain hospitals, the Royal London and St. James Charity, refused to consider it.

Disgruntled, Simon said, "I think we should have the paper published before presenting to the Royal College of Surgeons. We need to publish in *Lancet, Archiv für Klinische Chirurgie*, or the *Bulletin de l'Académie Imperiale de Médecine.* If we can get into one prestigious journal, the College will need to hear our data even though others will try to disprove our findings."

Rachel said spiritedly, "Let them try to disprove it. I know we and Semmelweis are in the right."

Rachel and Simon worked evenings to write their treatise on hypochlorite scrubbing, which included Semmelweis's data, their personal experience from London, and the data from the American Civil War.

They were almost finished with the paper when Rachel received a small packet from America postmarked eight weeks earlier. The packet contained a private note and a printed medical article entitled *A Report of Hospital Gangrene, Erysipelas and Pyemia*[30] by Dr. Middleton Goldsmith.

September 3, 1863
Dr. Rachel Romain
c/o St. James Charity Hospital
London, England
Dear Rachel,

I hope this letter finds you and your uncle safe and healthy in London. I learned only today from the note you left at the hotel that you and your uncle had been deported to England before I returned to Washington.

'Tis a shame as I so looked forward to seeing you again and learning more of your most unusual and remarkable life.

---

[30] Gangrene, erysipelas, and pyemia are all bacterial infections. At this time, bacteria was not thought to cause infections. Bacteria had been identified in the 1685 by Antoni van Leeuwenhoek using primitive microscopes.

I've enclosed a publication given to me by one of the surgeons in the Army of the Potomac. It was written last year by a surgeon, a Dr. Goldsmith, in the Army of the Cumberland in the Western Theater of war. I didn't understand much of the article, but the gist is that Dr. Goldsmith used bromine solution to treat gangrene and other infections with great success. Dr. Goldsmith could not explain why or what the bromine did to obtain such good results.

The surgeon who gave me the article said the publication is hogwash and not to be believed. No surgeon in the Army of the Potomac has adopted Goldsmith's methods. Something tells me you might think differently.

Anyway, I am sorry to have missed you. Unless we have a miracle, most believe this war may last another year or two. I know of no way you can correspond to me for as long as the Army of the Potomac remains on the move daily.

After the war, I'll need to return to Boston indefinitely to help restore our family's metal working business. Alas, we may never get to finish sharing our stories with each other.

Major Solomon Birch
Quartermaster, Army of the Potomac

Afterward, Rachel showed Simon the publication by Dr. Goldsmith but didn't mention her pining for Solomon Birch and the realization that she may never see him again.

"His results mirror ours," Simon said excitedly. "Perhaps bromine is less irritating than hypochlorite. It might be more acceptable to our colleagues."

Rachel was hesitant.

"It seems no one believes his data either," she said. "Goldsmith,[31] like us, gives no explanation as to why bromine works. Still, I believe we should include his results in our paper."

"Agreed," Simon said.

He submitted the paper to Europe's most prestigious medical journals and waited.

Following their war experience, Simon and Rachel became busier and busier as trauma surgeons and experts in amputation. They continued to use chlorite scrubbing, and their infection rate remained the best at both hospitals. Still, the other surgeons and all the nurses refused to adopt their methods.

By the spring of 1864, Simon had received rejections of their paper from each of the journals he'd submitted to. To make matters worse, Rachel had not heard from Solomon Birch again.

"My dear, I know it's upsetting, but you must see reason," Cynthia said gently as she and Rachel sat in the parlor after dinner. "The war continues. You cannot return to the United States, ever. Did you think this Solomon Birch would leave his family and business after the war to come here to be with you? That makes no sense."

"I suppose you're right," Rachel said.

Cynthia added, "You don't even know if he's made promises to another woman at home or, worse yet, has

---

[31] Goldsmith's publication describes his use of bromine aerosol to treat gangrene. His data showed a forty percent mortality rate for amputated patients diagnosed with gangrene. When bromine was applied to the wound, the mortality fell to three percent. He had no explanation for the success of bromine.

been injured or killed."

"Don't take away my hope," Rachel begged, suddenly impassioned. "He seemed genuinely interested in what I do. No other man I've yet met, other than Andrew, comes close. I thought fate might have brought us together. He told me that when we first met."

"I'll not take away your hope altogether," Cynthia said, "but you need to understand that Mr. Birch will very likely never come knocking on our door. Even if he did, he has no reason to stay here in England, and you can't even take one step into his country."

Rachel nodded, accepting the truth of Cynthia's statements.

After a moment of silence, Cynthia asked, "I could make introductions in case Mr. Birch doesn't respond?"

"Fine. I'll meet whomever you can dig up."

"I'm not 'digging up' anyone," Cynthia said with a raised voice.

"I'm sorry, Mum," Rachel said. "Go ahead and look. I don't have the strength to argue with you."

"We might find someone who appreciates your talent. I'd like nothing more than to find you a suitable husband and plan a proper wedding."

Rachel gave a subtle nod of acceptance and Cynthia exited the parlor.

"He'll respond," Rachel whispered to herself.

After reading the last journal denial, Simon spoke to Rachel and Cynthia over dinner. "I guess we'll try to present to the Royal College of Surgeons without having published. Perhaps our lecture will gain notice and allow publication."

Simon submitted his presentation to the annual meeting of the Royal College of Surgeons. In May, he learned the paper could be read on Monday, November 7, 1864, at 10 a.m.

As summer turned to fall, Rachel had still not heard from Solomon Birch. Through Cynthia and Simon, she'd been introduced to a number of available bachelors, all Jewish: James Rosenbloom, a barrister; Robèrt Razowsky, a Russian charge'-d'affaire; Warren Kifferstein, a successful wine merchant; and Roberto Tacher, a Moroccan businessman. Only Kifferstein asked to see Rachel again but she refused to answer his messages and gave as reasons to Cynthia: "too fat, too dull and too incredulous that I want to practice surgery."

"Shall we keep looking?" Cynthia asked.

"Of course. We may get lucky, yet," Rachel replied. "I've still not given up hopes of hearing from Mr. Birch."

As November neared, Simon and Rachel reviewed their data again and again. Simon practiced his talk, scheduled for thirty minutes with fifteen minutes allotted for discussion from the Fellows of the College.

"As much as I love you," Cynthia said privately to Simon, "public speaking is not your forte. You are reading verbatim in a monotone from your paper and don't hesitate between thoughts. There's no personality to it at all."

"I read the paper to Oscar Alanis," Simon said, "and he said the same. He told me the entire College will be asleep before I conclude."

"Might Rachel make the presentation?" Cynthia asked.

"No. It must be a member of the College. Sadly."

November rolled around and Simon's oratorical skills had not improved. In fact, he became so anxious even to practice that his presentation got worse. Cynthia and Rachel said nothing, knowing that criticism at this late date would only make the situation untenable.

Cynthia approached Simon after lunch two days before the meeting to try to calm his nerves. He had been practicing his talk all morning.

Simon lamented, "How is it that I can remove the

most difficult tumor and amputate a shattered leg, but cannot deliver a simple speech?"

"Many," Cynthia said, "without a farthing of talent in anything can deliver orations that lead men to war. You only need look at half of our Parliament."

Simon laughed and said, "Thank you."

"I need to get your mind off the presentation. We're going out tonight with Sir Archibald and his new wife, Celeste, to celebrate Guy Fawkes Day[32]," Cynthia said. "Archie has been the most wonderful friend since retiring."

"Where are we going? I'd like to return at a reasonable hour to practice my talk a bit more," Simon said.

"Absolutely not. You need to clear your head before tackling the talk again. We're going to Battersea Park," Cynthia said. "The fireworks are second only to Lewes. We'll sample the vendors' fare. Archie went last year and said it would take your mind off the talk. He tried something called 'fish and chips' for the first time and can't wait to try them again."

"Sounds disgusting," Simon said.

Simon's stomach pains started at two a.m., the vomiting at two-thirty. Cynthia and Rachel did their best to stem the symptoms with laudanum for the pain and licorice root and angostura bitters for the nausea.

"He has no fever or diarrhea yet," Rachel said. "I don't believe this is a recurrence of typhoid, though of course, it's worrying."

---

[32] *Guy Fawkes Day has been celebrated in England on November 5th each year since the early 1600s and celebrates a failed plot to blow up the English Parliament by Catholic Papists. Bonfires, fireworks and hanging Catholic dolls in effigy were common until the mid-19th century when anti-Catholic sentiment died down. The holiday kept the fireworks, bonfires and added feasting to the celebration, which continues to this day.*

A loud knock on the door startled everyone. Sharron answered the door and brought a note up to Simon's bedroom for Cynthia to read.

"It seems," Cynthia said, "that Sir Archibald is suffering from an ill stomach too, with vomiting, nausea and stomach pain. He's taking laudanum and bitters, with little relief."

Cynthia clapped a hand to her forehead. "You two were the only ones to eat the 'fish and chips'! I think I've identified the source of the malaise."

Simon could only nod.

"I'd agree. I'll send a note back to Sir Archibald's house," Rachel said. "The illness will likely run its course in two or three days. We need only to keep them hydrated with tea, honey and water."

By Sunday night, the vomiting had subsided, although the sour stomach persisted. Still dehydrated, Simon had difficulty getting out of the bed. Rachel felt a rush of love for her uncle; he looked so frail, and had been through so much.

"What cruel fate," Simon said. "I was to deliver our paper in the morning to the College."

"Will they allow me to deliver it?" Rachel asked, knowing the answer.

"No," Simon moaned. "Worse yet, Sir Archibald was going to introduce me. I assume he's no better than I."

Cynthia said, "I received a note from Celeste that he is improving but too out of sorts to attend the College meeting tomorrow."

Rachel shrugged and said, "Not to worry. I will go and tell the moderator our dilemma. Perhaps they will let me present. If not, another year will pass."

Chapter Nineteen
Post Hoc

On Monday morning, Rachel took the paper in hand and went to the Burlington House in Piccadilly, the site of the annual meeting of the Royal College of Surgeons. She arrived at 8:30 a.m., a half hour before the first scheduled talk and ninety minutes before Simon's appointed time.

She found Mr. Richard Port, the President of the College, instructing attendants in the arrangement of chairs in the great hall. Port turned to greet Rachel.

"Mr. Port," Rachel said briskly. "We've met. I'm Doctor Rachel Romain, the surgeon at St. James Charity and the niece of Mr. Simon Romain."

"Yes, I remember you," Port said. "What can I do for you?"

"First, let me tell you how much I enjoy your book on the *Principles of Surgery.* I refer to it often and am always edified by your experience," Rachel lied, knowing Port to be a blowhard.

"Thank you," Port said, with a condescending bow of his head.

"I'm afraid Simon and Sir Archibald Leach have contracted food poisoning. They went together to Battersea Park for the Guy Fawkes celebration on Saturday eve and ate 'fish and chips' from a food vendor. Both have been in distress since then. Neither is well enough to attend today's meeting."

"Oh, my. That's unfortunate," Port said. "Many of our members had decided opinions on Simon's work. Like a pride of lions circling their prey, I would think."

Rachel took a deep breath.

"Might I deliver the paper? I am the co-author and Simon's research partner; I was in the United States performing surgeries for the entire duration of our research," Rachel said. "I know that only Fellows of the College are allowed to present, but it would be a shame to allow a huge gap in the program."

Port scratched his bald head, thinking, and appeared momentarily speechless.

"Besides," Rachel said hurriedly, "the lions will be hungry and why not allow them to feast while they have me at their disposal?"

Port laughed but continued to think of his options. "That would squelch their hunger for only a few hours. An Irish surgeon presents at 3 p.m. with a bizarre procedure for hemorrhoids. I might delay the feast till then."

"Please, Mr. Port. I believe that under the circumstances it might be acceptable for me to make the delivery. If the body of the College decides they won't hear from me, then so be it. Hopefully, you can make the introduction as Sir Archibald is also indisposed. You then might make a case for me to be allowed to speak."

"I can try," Port said doubtfully.

"If they anticipate a feeding frenzy, they might well let me present."

Port coughed.

"You've got spine, I'll admit that much," he said. "But two hundred Fellows against one female are not good odds. I expect invited guests in the gallery above to take the side of the Fellows as well. Are you sure you want to present in these conditions?"

"Why not?" Rachel responded without hesitation. "A single elephant, even a female one, can challenge a pride of lions."

Port laughed again. "I would presume so, although I had you pegged as a gazelle?"

"No," Rachel said. "A gazelle would run from danger. I won't."

"Touché, Dr. Romain," Port said. "Then all I've heard of you seems true. Make sure you speak loudly so the back of the room can hear clearly. Nothing angers the Fellows more than not being able to hear."

"I will yell, if necessary."

"Are there any members of the College you wish me not to call on?" Port asked.

"Perhaps only Sir John Minkove. He and Simon don't see eye to eye on a few things and I've defended Simon."

Port's jovial face grew contemplative.

"As the knighted past president of the College, it would be hard not to call on Sir John if he raises his hand. Let's pray he doesn't."

The 9 a.m. presentation by Mr. Nathan Tross of Newcastle-Upon-Tyne on his two years of experience using a mechanical device with a bellow to deliver chloroform met with laughter and derision. When a Fellow suggested the bellow reminded him of a miniature accordion, the entire room erupted in laughter.

At 10 a.m., Mr. Port ascended to the podium to introduce Mr. Simon Romain's paper on *The Use of Hypochlorite Scrubbing to Reduce the Incidence of Putrefaction.* Many of the Fellows leaned left or right to a compatriot and whispered something, both smiling.

"Unfortunately," Port went on, "Sir Archibald Leach, who was to make the introduction, and Mr. Simon Romain, whose research was to be presented, have fallen ill with food poisoning. Rather than waste an hour, his niece, Dr. Rachel Romain, the surgeon at St. James Charity, has consented to present the paper."

Immediately, a few members stamped their feet on the floor chanting, "No women, no women ..."

Port raised his hand to quiet the crowd. "Dr. Romain is not a member of the College for obvious reasons. Still, she has consented to deliver the paper and accept criticism, without prejudice of her fair sex. I see no reason why she should not be allowed to speak. After all, we are learned men."

Although Rachel had never presented a paper in front of her peers, she knew the material better than anyone, including Simon. She had decided that morning as she perused Simon's speech that she would deliver their findings without notes.

Rachel took the podium, expecting some to leave for no reason other than she was a woman, ill-suited to be in a man's position. However, the Fellows of the College had not been prepared for someone as young and attractive as she. At that point, she had every Fellow's attention. Without hesitation, she began with a strong and confident voice.

"Mr. Port, Fellows of the Royal College of Surgeons, thank you for allowing me to present Mr. Simon Romain's research on the prevention of wound infection using sodium hypochlorite solution scrubs. Our research is based on the finding of Dr. Ignaz Semmelweis, a Hungarian obstetrician ..."

Rachel took the full thirty minutes of allotted time presenting Semmelweis's findings, Goldsmith's usage of bromine, and ended with their results from the Civil War battlefields.

"...Simon and I performed two-hundred-twenty-seven amputations within forty-eight hours of injury and where hypochlorite scrubbing and isolation had been used with a minimum of seven days of follow up. The other surgeons, Confederate and Union, had seven-hundred-twelve patients followed for at least seven days as well. Our infection rate was five-point-two percent. The other surgeons had a twenty-point-three percent infection rate."

Rachel paused before her summary.

"I will be the first to admit that neither Simon nor I know why Semmelweis's and our results are so significantly positive. We believe the cause of infection comes from the skin or wounds of the injured patient and is then transmitted to others from the surgeon's and nurse's hands or equipment. Thank you again for the privilege of allowing me to present Mr. Simon Romain's research. I am happy to answer any questions."

Within seconds, a sea of hands materialized. Mr. Port returned to the podium to introduce Fellows to ask questions of Rachel.

"Young Mr. Kennedy," Port said, pointing to a Fellow near the front, who the day before had been elected to the Royal College of Surgeons.

The man stood and announced himself. "Mr. Robert Kennedy, Jr., Belfast. Dr. Romain, you are going against two thousand years of dictum that infection is airborne. We all know it is miasma. For that matter, I still don't fathom how Edward Jenner has duped everyone in this country with his cowpox farce. Why waste your and our time with this rubbish?"

"A good question, Mr. Kennedy," Rachel said. "For millions of years, everyone in the world believed the earth was flat. Then Magellan circled the globe to prove once and for all that the earth is round. I cannot tell you why with certainty, but scrubbing with hypochlorite reduced the incidence of infection and death. That is undeniable. With this knowledge, we can save more lives."

Kennedy scoured the crowd mulishly. "I for one," he declared, "will not be scrubbing anything."

A large percentage of Fellows stood with fists raised, yelling, "Here, here."

When the yelling stopped, Rachel responded. "Mr. Kennedy, you must do what you believe to be in the best interest of your patients. But, if you get on a ship heading in any direction from Ireland, I sincerely hope you don't fall over the edge of the earth into the abyss."

A few laughed at Rachel's bon mot, but many crossed their arms and shook heads at an outsider trying to ridicule a Fellow of the College.

Mr. Port leaned to Rachel and mumbled, "Be careful. You could make the lions attack. He pointed to a young Fellow in the back. "I'm sorry, I don't know your name."

The man stood. "Mr. Joseph Lister, Glasgow."[33]

"Your comment?" Port asked.

"I think the Romains should be commended for tackling a subject for which we have no answers. Why do patients upon whom we perform the perfect procedure still die at an alarming rate? The Romains, unfortunately, have two issues that need solving. First, they can't answer why their solution works. Secondly, hypochlorite is toxic and difficult to work with. But we shouldn't diminish their efforts. I, for one, will think on their work and try to solve their concerns."

"Thank you, Mr. Lister," Rachel said.

Hands remained raised in the hall and Port pointed to another Fellow. "Mr. Brown."

The man stood. "Mr. Chester Brown, Manchester. You say that you and your uncle went to the rebellious states and did this research in the middle of a civil war. The difference between bravery and stupidity is often a very thin line. How do we know you actually did all this work? What proof is there other than your word? How do we know you weren't merely playing Cowboys and Indians this whole time like my seven-year-old grandson?"

When the laughter died down, Rachel responded. "You have Simon Romain's word, and my own, and the log books from our research. That is all I can offer," Rachel said.

"Jews have been known to stretch the truth," Brown said.

A number of the Fellows nodded heads in agreement. The antisemitic comment caught Rachel by surprise, and her cheeks flushed with anger. Just as the laughter died down, a loud, clear voice from the visitor's

---

[33] Joseph Lister: A few years later, Lister revolutionized surgery by using Louis Pasteur's findings that microorganisms are the cause of wound infection. Lister introduced antiseptics (carbolic acid) to fight infections, transforming patient outcomes and laying the foundation upon which modern healthcare practices are built.

gallery turned heads.

"I believe that I can vouch for Dr. Romain's presence on the battlefield and her research," said a voice from the rear of the gallery.

Rachel, Mr. Port, Mr. Brown, and the entirety of the Fellows looked up into the gallery to find the voice.

Port asked, "Sir, who might you be?"

"My name is Solomon Birch. I am a retired Colonel in the Army of the Potomac, at present under the command of General Ulysses S. Grant."

The crowd of Fellows erupted in surprised murmurs.

"Come down, Colonel Birch," Port called, "and tell us why you are here and what you know."

Solomon descended from the gallery to join a stunned and speechless Rachel and a curious Mr. Richard Port. Rachel stepped back and allowed Solomon and Port to take center stage. She stared at Solomon, unable to believe it was really him.

"What brings an American army officer to Britain?" Port asked.

"I served my country for three years in the battlefield, promoted to colonel, and was discharged honorably," Solomon said. "My family has been in the metal works business for decades. We've approached Martin Weitz and Company, a noted British surgical instrument manufacturer, whom I believe you all know, to begin a joint venture on both sides of the Atlantic. I arrived in town yesterday and was invited here by Sir John Minkove."

"How is it that you know Dr. Romain?" Port asked.

Solomon said, "I must tell it on the whole. On May 1st last year, I was a quartermaster for the Army of the Potomac's XI Corps as we fought Robert E. Lee at the Battle of Chancellorsville in the State of Virginia. The battle was intense and we were being beaten rather soundly by the Confederates.

"At noon on the first day of battle, I was leading a

group of wagons attempting to deliver musket balls and powder to our men. I took a wrong turn. When I tried to turn about, I was shot in the hand and knocked off my wagon, landing on my shoulder and head and rendered unconscious.

"When I awoke, I found myself in the back of a Confederate ambulance with six other injured men, including one other severely injured Union soldier. My hand had been bandaged with dirty linen and blood was seeping through. I was dumped into a tent and chained to a post with guards posted outside.

"The other Union soldier was unconscious and in the throes of death with gaping wounds of the chest and abdomen. He stopped breathing an hour after arriving. I was given no water or food and no one had examined my hand. In the early hours of the morning, a young woman entered my tent and identified herself as Dr. Rachel Romain, a surgeon. She spoke with a decidedly British accent. My first thought was that she was a young, ill-trained British nurse, forced beyond her competency by a lack of real surgeons. I was wrong."

Solomon had garnered every Fellow's compete attention and he continued the story.

"She had the guard take me to a farm house turned into a makeshift hospital where she examined my wounds. My little finger was gone and half the ring finger hung by a sliver of tissue. She said she needed to remove the dangling ring finger portion and clean the stump of my little finger. She retrieved an assistant who put me to sleep with chloroform."

Solomon held up his injured hand to show the missing digit and a half.

"Shortly after I awoke in the morning, Dr. Romain returned and changed my bandage. We both agreed that I would likely be sent to a Confederate prison camp. That was the last time I spoke with Dr. Romain."

"What a hellish situation," Port said. "How did you manage to escape the prison camp?"

Solomon continued. "The Union had captured a Confederate Brigadier General earlier that day. By some measure of incredible luck, I was swapped for the General. From what others have told me since, if I had been in any other Confederate hospital and sent to a prison camp, I would not have had my hand seen for days or even weeks, and infection of the hand would most likely have occurred. I wouldn't be here today."

"An amazing story, Colonel Birch," Brown said from the floor, "but what proof do you have of her research?"

"I returned to service in time for the Battle of Gettysburg that July. As the battle turned in our favor and Robert E. Lee and the rebels began their retreat, I learned that Dr. Romain was the only Confederate surgeon who had refused to leave her post and had kept working until all the ether, chloroform, bandages and sutures in her hospital had been exhausted. Still, she didn't leave. She was captured by our cavalry and swore to the commanding Union officer she would continue to do her research and not try to escape until all the men, Union and Confederate, were treated. The officer supplied Dr. Romain with the equipment and drugs she needed, plus additional surgeons. As quartermaster, I helped gather those materials. Dr. Romain worked for another week until she was formally arrested."

"Dr. Romain was arrested? Tell me more?" Port asked.

"She spent days in a makeshift tent stockade outside Gettysburg then was transferred to a prison in Washington for trial. At trial, she admitted to having entered the Confederate States illegally and aided the rebellion, but she did it only after the Union Surgeon General had refused to let her do her research for the North. She felt the research was too important not to be done. In total, she spent twelve days in jail. The judge found her guilty and sentenced her to the time already spent. So she was set free. Days later, her uncle, Mr.

Simon Romain, still in the South and recovering from typhoid, was exchanged for a captured Confederate surgeon. Once the exchange had been completed, she and her uncle were deported, as undesirables, back to Britain."

"Their research. What proof do you have?" Brown insisted.

"Apparently, at her trial and under oath, she presented the logbooks and spoke at length on her research, detailing every aspect. The courtroom was packed with Union soldiers whom she had treated. I believe it was her fervent desire to prove her theories that convinced the judge that Dr. Romain was not an enemy of the state and didn't deserve to spend additional time in prison."

Port brought Rachel back to the center and asked, "Quite the escapade, Dr.Romain. Is it all true as Colonel Birch has described?"

"Yes. Every word," Rachel said. "I had no idea Mr. Birch would be in England, let alone here at the Royal College's meeting. An amazing coincidence."

Port turned to the Fellows and asked, "Any more questions of Dr. Romain?"

A flurry of hand raising occurred until a member of the College in the front row stood. All the raised hands in the audience fell immediately. Port had no option but to call on the standing man.

"Sir John."

"Sir John Minkove, London. Dr. Romain, congratulations on you and your uncle's heroic but misbegotten attempt to prove, in my opinion, a dodgy theory."

A low-toned groan erupted from the Fellows. Sir John continued. "Your proof, as does Dr. Semmelweiss', uses the *post hoc ergo propter hoc* fallacy.

I've read Dr. Semmelweis's work. The *Gazette médicale de Paris* journal dismissed it on those grounds. If you had gone to medical school and then completed a proper education and surgical training, you'd know and understand the *post hoc ergo propter hoc* fallacy.[34]"

The gallery of Fellows, nodding agreement in unison, responded with "Here, here," and started talking to each other.

Standing beside Solomon, Rachel had no clue what the *post hoc ergo propter hoc* fallacy meant and didn't know what to say. Solomon turned to see Rachel's eyes searching, at a loss for words.

As the Fellows jeered noisily, Solomon leaned over and whispered, "You assume one thing caused another only because the hypochlorite scrub preceded the absence of infection. That is not proof."

Rachel nodded understanding and mumbled, "Thanks."

"*Illegitimi non carborundum est*," Solomon added in a whisper.

"Huh?"

"Latin for 'Don't let the bastards grind you down.'"

Rachel smiled as Port held his hands up to silence the Fellows, then turned and asked Rachel, "How do you respond to Sir John's criticism?"

Rachel responded in a strong, convincing tone. "Thank you, Sir John, for your opinion. As physicians and surgeons, we all attend patients who declare, 'I ate fish at supper last night and got sick, so it must be the fish.' The perfect example of the *post hoc ergo propter hoc* fallacy."

Heads bobbed among the Fellows as most nodded agreement.

"We all know blaming the fish is conjecture. It could have been the pudding or cornbread or none of those things."

---

[34] *Post hoc ergo propter hoc fallacy*: literally translated it means "after this, therefore because of this." The fact that X happened before Y, doesn't prove X caused Y.

The Fellows smiled and nodded agreement again.

"Simon and I performed two-hundred-twenty-seven amputations with hypochlorite scrubs to achieve a bit more than a five percent infection rate. The other surgeons had seven hundred twelve patients without scrubbing and had a twenty-three percent infection rate. If I serve nine-hundred and thirty-nine Fellows of the Royal College of Surgeons dinner, and seven hundred twelve have fish, pudding and cornbread and all get sick whilst the two-hundred twenty seven who had mutton, pudding and cornbread did not, then the fish would seem the culprit. It's simple logic."

The Fellows nod once again.

"Sir John, you have a right to your own opinion on infection, as does every Fellow in the hall. But I do not have an opinion."

Rachel paused, keeping the Fellows, now curious, on the edge of their seats. "I have data, hard data, and you do not have that."

Sir John stood and exclaimed, "Who do you think you are?" He then marched out of the hall. Half the Fellows followed Sir John out and started chattering to each other outside the hall.

Port sidled close to Rachel and said, "You've done it now and wounded one of the black-maned lions. They will devour you if you stay. Time to step down."

Port stepped to the front. "Thank you, Dr. Romain for presenting your uncle's research. Our next speaker, Mr. Robert Philip, from Wimbledon, will present on his novel approach to hernias."

As Rachel and Solomon exited the stage, Solomon said, "I'm eager to speak with you, but best we act only cordial. They mustn't think it's a plot. Minkove is a close friend of Martin Weitz. If possible, I'll find you when I'm done with business."

Solomon showed Rachel his repaired hand but then returned immediately to the gallery. Rachel stood frozen to the side until a few Fellows came to congratulate her on the presentation, including Mr. Joseph Lister. Rachel ascended the gallery and took a seat far away from Solomon.

She tried to concentrate on the speakers but in anticipation of seeing Solomon again, her stomach churned. She then remembered the offhand remark she had made to him about manufacturing surgical instruments so they would have reason to meet once more. Was he here only to see me? Was it merely a business venture? She closed her eyes and hoped, 'Let it be me.'

Rachel laughed to herself. She had just passed her thirtieth birthday but her anxieties were those of a fourteen-year-old. Still, she couldn't concentrate and left the hall after two lectures to return to St. James Charity.

Chapter Twenty
Solent #2

At dinner, Rachel told Cynthia and Simon the saga of her presentation and rescue by Solomon Birch, whom she remembered had studied philosophy and logic at Harvard University. "He said he would try to seek me out after completing his business in London. We parted ways without even a handshake. I so wanted to find out why he was in London."

"I'm sure he'll call," Cynthia said.

"I hope so," Rachel said. "At the trial in Washington, he disappeared without a word."

"More importantly, how was the paper received?" Simon asked.

"Important to whom?" Cynthia asked.

Rachel laughed. "I'm fine, Mum. A few Fellows congratulated me. A Mr. Joseph Lister was most cordial. Besides that, I don't know. I suppose many of the Fellows didn't want to show support whilst Sir John Minkove remained out of sorts."

"Good," Simon said. "I hope he remains that way. Stubborn as an ox."

Rachel looked to Simon, "'Tis a shame that you and Sir John have argued about using hemp as a suture material. I believe most think silk and gut are better choices today but Sir John has a problem admitting that he might have been wrong. It didn't help me today."

"I agree with Solomon," Simon said. "Showing too much friendship to Mr. Birch could anger some Fellows and suggest a plot. Speaking personally, however, I cannot wait to meet him."

"I'd have to agree with Simon on this," Cynthia said.

Simon added, "You've made an enemy of Sir John, and he holds the strings to many puppets in the Royal College. I know for a fact he consults with the Weitz Company on surgical tool design."

"Mr. Birch mentioned the same but I didn't know that. Anyway, I had to defend our research," Rachel said.

"It might put your Mr. Birch in a squeeze with Martin Weitz if Sir John has his ear," Simon said.

"Hopefully not. I don't know what 'I'll try to find you after my business' means,'" Rachel said.

"It means," Cynthia said, "that he won't see you until he's done with Sir John and Weitz. Be prepared that Weitz and Sir John may stay with him 'til he's boarded a ship home."

"Don't even say that," Rachel gasped.

Two days went by and Rachel had not received even a note from Solomon.

"Do you think he's upset with me and won't call or even send a note?" Rachel asked Cynthia. "I hope he hasn't returned to Boston already. What should I do?"

"You wait, my dear."

The next evening Cynthia showed Rachel, who remained in a funk, an invitation she'd received for a charity gala for retired Royal Navy veterans.

"I have no interest in such a thing. I've given donations to the Royal Navy but never enough to be invited," Rachel said.

Cynthia smiled and said, "Look closer. Look at who chairs the event, Lady Linda Weitz and Countess Olivia Lipson-Drayer."

Rachel took the invitation and scanned it. "What does it mean?"

Cynthia said, "Olivia must be working with Lady Weitz to prepare the gala. Perhaps Olivia might play Cupid for you if you're still on her good side. It's worth a try as long as Sir John doesn't get wind of it. What did you call those things -a long shot?"

Rachel sent a note to Olivia, suggesting a luncheon meeting as soon as possible. Another day went by without a word from Solomon, but she received an invitation from Olivia to meet at Brown's Hotel at noon the next day – the same restaurant as their first meeting.

Rachel arrived at eleven-thirty and notified the maître d' that she would wait in the hotel lounge. At noon, the maître d' escorted Rachel to the countess's table. Following a curtsy, Rachel sat.

"You look well," Olivia said

"Thank you," Rachel said, noting Olivia's, smooth complexion, tailored dress, and fashionable style of braided bun and side braids. "As do you. I love your hair. I don't think I could do that."

"It takes work and time, something I imagine you don't have much of with your workload."

"I pray you have enough time for me to catch up with you," Rachel said.

"I hear nothing but good things about you. Surgeon at St. James Charity. Such a noble cause," Olivia said.

"Never a day has gone by when I don't have a thought of Andrew," Rachel said, changing subjects. "He'd be a famous barrister by now."

"Yes. I think of him often too," Olivia said sadly. "But I don't suppose you've called me here to reminisce."

Rachel winced, aware that this was the first time she'd contacted Olivia since Andrew's death only because she wanted something. Then again, Olivia had never been shy about hiding what she wanted. Rachel gathered her resolve.

"That's true, I wish to ask your help with something, but it's a long story."

"Oh. I love intrigue. We have all lunch to get through it and I've heard you've been abroad on some adventure," Olivia said with a smile.

Rachel shook her head and thought, 'she knows everything.' Regardless, Rachel began, and soon her story was in full swing. "Simon and I snuck into Virginia on a gunrunner to escape the Northern states blockade.

We were there to do research on wound infection with the Confederate Army and — "

"— Already a good story, if nothing else, " Olivia interrupted.

As the soup dishes disappeared and the prime rib and scalloped potatoes appeared, Rachel got to treating Solomon Birch after he was injured. Later, as the prime rib was taken away, Rachel told how she had seen Solomon for only a few seconds at her trial but then he had disappeared without a word.

Then Solomon blindsided Rachel at the Royal College of Surgeons meeting at the expense of Sir John Minkove. She learned Solomon was working with Martin Weitz to make surgical instruments. Lastly, Rachel countered and angered Sir John's logic with logic of her own causing him to rush from the auditorium.

Rachel ended her lengthy story with, "Mr. Birch said he'd get in touch with me when his business is done. It's been three days and I've heard nothing. I believe he's interested in me, so his silence is a mystery," Rachel lamented.

"I'm confused. How do I fit into this?" Olivia asked.

"It's a bit convoluted. My uncle, Simon and Sir John Minkove have had disagreements, still not resolved. You are working with Lady Weitz. I know Sir John is close with the Weitzes, so perhaps Mr. Birch can't approach me with them hovering. I'm afraid Martin Weitz will force Solomon back on a ship to Boston without me being able to learn his true intentions."

"So you want me to extricate Solomon Birch from the Weitzes," Olivia said, "and sneak him off somewhere so you can meet in secret?"

"Yes. If it's possible," Rachel said.

"Hmm. I've met this Solomon Birch at the Weitz's manor. He, Martin and Sir John were working on diagrams of strange contraptions, as far as I could see. Quite tall and handsome actually."

"Am I mad for asking this favor of you?"

"You pulled off the Cowes Regatta in disguise, which to this day, people still talk about. I believe I still owe you. I would also like to see you find happiness again."

Rachel beamed with gratitude.

Olivia added, "Sir John believes he is God's gift to man. The fact you one-upped him in front of the College of Surgeons is reason enough to help you."

The two women shared a conspiratorial laugh.

"Linda Weitz is as perceptive as I," Olivia said, growing serious. "I'd need to do something unplanned to make it happen without raising suspicion. I'm at her house tomorrow. If Mr. Birch is present, I will see what I can concoct. This is quite exciting, actually."

Rachel and Olivia finished their lunch. When they stood, Rachel embraced Olivia and said, "Thank you."

"I'll write you a note as to my success. It may not work out," Olivia cautioned her.

"I understand. But I will be on pins and needles, waiting."

Rachel had trouble concentrating all the next day, apart from four hours she spent in surgery at St. James Charity. Cynthia acted as scrub nurse for her that day.

"I'm glad surgery allows me to focus," Rachel said, "no matter what else is going on in my life. I haven't thought of Solomon or Olivia since the incision."

"Simon says the same," Cynthia said. "Must be something inherited from his side of the family."

"Is that a thing?" Rachel asked, stopping and looking up at Cynthia from the task at hand. "I wonder if Solomon focuses so well."

Cynthia laughed, handing Rachel a suture. "You lost focus, my dear. Close the incision."

Rachel placed the first suture into the lowest edge of the skin incision and tied a knot.

Cynthia cut the tied suture and said, "You resemble your father and uncle in many ways. For me, when I have something on my mind that bothers me, I think of nothing else. When we were newlyweds, before we had Sharron to cook for us, I burned more roasts than you can imagine."

When Rachel arrived home that evening, a note waited for her. She found Cynthia and read the note aloud.

> Rachel,
>
> It's been far too long since you've been on the Solent. No races or competition this time, just a couple days cruising on the Lipson family yacht, *The Biscuit.* Depending on November weather, we might head east this time and put in at Brighton.
>
> This Saturday at the yacht club in Southampton. Leave port at 0800, weather permitting.
>
> Olivia

Rachel smiled, put the note down and looked to Cynthia.

"She doesn't mention Solomon," Cynthia said cautiously.

"It's a coded message," Rachel said. "She wouldn't have penned this note if Solomon wasn't going to be there."

Rachel left London on the Friday evening train to Southampton. As her cab passed the Canute Castle Hotel, her heart sank at the memory of Andrew making love to her. She wouldn't stay there this time, knowing those memories could not be suppressed. Through tears, she thought to herself, 'Andrew would be happy that I'm looking for love again. It's been time enough.'

Rachel checked into the Star Hotel, which had seen better days, although the new iron grating across the front of the hotel above the carriage arch gave it a bit of class. The knot in her stomach grew worse with worry about the day to come. She barely touched her supper and slept little that night.

The next morning, Rachel, in an overcoat and her

linen sailing togs, left the hotel at 6:30 a.m., toting her sea bag. She knew the ship's crew would already be working to get *The Biscuit* ready. Fortune favored them, with the sun out, mild winds, and temperatures in the 60s. This time, she would board a Lipson family boat as a woman.

Approaching the dock, she heard the six bells of the morning watch. *The Biscuit* was a magnificent 100-foot, 110-ton, double masted gaff schooner built for comfort as a private sailing yacht.

Olivia had forewarned the crew of Rachel's presence and explained to them the legend of the girl on the *Glory B* in the Cowes Week Regatta.

"All hands, attention. Royalty on board," shouted a seaman. The crew stood to attention and saluted Rachel.

"Stop it, men. I was but a lowly cabin boy," Rachel said with a smile. "Well, maybe not."

Rachel drew honest laughter from the six seamen on deck. As she introduced herself to each, Olivia boarded the ship.

Before Rachel could curtsy, the custom before a countess, Olivia wrapped her in a hug. "You needn't curtsy to me unless we're at some official function. I booked rooms at the Royal Yacht club for Martin Weitz and Mr. Birch. I told Martin to deliver Mr. Birch here not before half eight,[35] the first bell of the forenoon watch, then Martin will return to London."

"Does Mr. Weitz even know what the forenoon watch is?' Rachel asked.

"None whatsoever."

"Weitz isn't coming on board?"

"No," Olivia said. "He was only too happy to have his house and Linda to himself for a couple of days. I knew my ploy would work when Linda confided that neither Martin nor Sir John could stomach yachting. I'll deliver Mr. Birch back to Martin at the end of the cruise."

"What should I do now?" Rachel asked. "Might I stay

---

[35] Half eight: 18th century English idiom for half past the hour and still used today.

on deck? I don't think Mr. Weitz knows me."

"Can't take that chance. He might have been at your presentation to the Fellows."

"That's possible," Rachel agreed. "I slept not at all last night. Not like me to worry about a man."

Olivia laughed. "Martin might arrive sooner than I instructed so he can catch the early train back to London. I'd suggest going below deck to the Captain's quarters and staying there until you're at sea. You can stow your bag there as well."

"Where will you stay?" Rachel asked.

"I'm not going," Olivia said.

"You're not?" Rachel asked, genuinely surprised.

"No, I've got some redecorating to do in our Southampton house. Besides, I'd be in the way. I'll wait for Mr. Weitz to leave before you shove off. You and Solomon can stay in the Captain's quarters."

"It'll be our secret," Rachel said.

"Of course," Olivia said, with a sparkle in her eye. "Like the night you spent with Andrew at the Canute Castle after the regatta."

"You knew?" Rachel cried.

"Of course. Andrew wasn't with the other men that night," Olivia said. "Doesn't take a fool to figure it out."

"When I lied to you at lunch about my virginity, you knew?"

"Yes," Olivia said. "But I was wrong to accuse you of offering sexual favors. It was none of my business."

"You are, indeed, a most remarkable woman," Rachel said.

"As are you," Olivia said. "Now go below and stow your gear."

Rachel went below deck to the captain's quarters, dropped her tote bag on the floor and removed her shoes. She heard the eight bells ending the morning watch and the beginning of the forenoon watch. Solomon would be coming soon.

The portholes provided a decent view of the

gangplank but she decided not to risk being seen by Weitz. Exhausted from worry and lack of sleep, Rachel laid down on the bed to wait. The gentle rocking of the boat put her to sleep in an instant.

An hour later, Rachel awoke with a start to feel the ship swaying beneath her. *The Biscuit* had left port. Rachel jumped off the bed and was halfway to the door when she heard a voice.

"You were sound asleep and looked too peaceful to awaken."

Rachel wheeled around and found Solomon sitting on a bedside chair, smiling. Wearing a business suit, he looked out of place.

"I didn't sleep at all last night," Rachel said, her heart pounding. "The rocking of the boat got to me."

"I enjoyed sitting there," Solomon said, standing, "just watching you. I know you as a whirling dervish, so seeing you so calm was a treat."

"Were you surprised to find me here?"

"I thought Martin Weitz had tired of me and asked the Countess to take me off his hands, which I thought excessive. I was interested to see how yachting here differs from New England but I expected to be bored after a day. When the Countess saw that Martin had departed the dock, she pointed to the Captain's quarters. When I turned back she was walking down the gangplank."

"I was hiding here to prevent Mr. Weitz from seeing me."

"A wise move," Solomon said. "I entered the quarters and thought I was dreaming. How did you arrange this? No easy feat, I can imagine, unless you are also best friends with the countess."

"The countess and I have more in common than you might guess," Rachel said. "So much to talk about. What are you to wear? That suit won't work."

"Of course. I've brought loose pants and shirt and hat. I can't wait to get out of these shoes and feel the deck under my bare feet."

Rachel smiled and closed on Solomon. He was taller than she remembered. Still unsure how Solomon felt about her, she stopped and held her breath, hoping for a clue or a sign.

"I've missed you so....," Solomon said with glassy eyes.

Rachel looked up at the clear message written on his face.

"...More than you'll ever know. I play our meeting in Chancellorsville over and over in my head."

Rachel, no longer unsure, took his hands, stood on her toes and kissed him on the lips.

Solomon, surprised by the kiss, stood back a step. "I think this might be the best two days of my life."

"I hope so."

"The man who carried my bag told me you're something of a legend but wouldn't tell me more."

Rachel giggled.

"We've so much to talk of. I know so little of you and you of me. Quick, get into something comfortable and I'll meet you on the deck."

Solomon appeared on deck ten minutes later in sailing togs and a heavy sweater. He asked the closest seaman where Rachel had gone. The seaman pointed up to the top of the mainmast. There sat Rachel, one foot on a ratline and the other on a spreader looking back at Southampton.

"Ahoy," Solomon yelled up, "may I join you?"

"I'd like that!"

Solomon climbed the ratlines to reach Rachel. Standing a ratline below Rachel, they stood nose to nose. "I have two brothers who wouldn't dare climb to the top of the mast."

"When you first told me that you and your family are boaters, I was certain that fate brought us together. I was raised on a merchant ship."

"I need to hear it all," Solomon said.

Rachel pointed to the horizon and told Solomon about her father, the Captain, and her former life as Ray. Solomon listened intently.

"I want to know more, everything about you and your fascinating life," he said. "And we've only two days!"

"What if I don't want you to leave?" Rachel asked.

"I must return to Boston. Much depends on what deal I can strike with Weitz and Company," Solomon said.

"You know I can't come with you. I'm an undesirable."

"Something else for me to work on at home."

"Let's go down and we'll explore *The Biscuit.* I've not seen her before," Rachel said.

"Yes," Solomon said, then leaned over and kissed her.

The winds began to gust wildly that day so Rachel suggested they stay in the Solent, protected from the wind, rather than venture into the English Channel. Alongside the Chief Mate, Solomon and Rachel took turns at the helm. With the seamen, they helped raise the jib and tightened the sails. Afterwards, they lunched with the crew on deck while Solomon told stories of his experiences in the Civil War.

In the early afternoon, they sat alone in the fore of the yacht to talk. Haltingly, Rachel told of Andrew and the Cowes Week regatta and their short engagement.

"That explains your relationship with the countess. I'm sorry for your loss," Solomon said. "I know I would have liked Andrew as well."

"And what of you?" Rachel asked. "Have you loved before?"

"When I left Harvard, I got engaged," Solomon said, taking one of Rachel's hands in his, "to the younger sister of my best friend. I'd known her all my life. Ever since we were nine and ten, her parents and mine had been certain we'd marry."

"What happened?"

"She was sweet, smart and pretty, but frightened of everything. After one short cruise on our yacht on the Cape in a bit of a wind storm, she swore she'd never step foot on a boat again. Even traveling by train to New York or Maine required spirits to calm her nerves. As much as I cared for her and her family, even her brother told me secretly he didn't think I'd be happy. When I went off to war in '61, she was certain I'd die. I called off our engagement and haven't met anyone since."

"No one?" Rachel asked.

"No one 'til you," Solomon said. "I wanted the war to end for no other reason than to be able to see you and ask how you felt about me. Honestly, I had given up hope."

"How was it that you came to seek out Mr. Weitz?"

"It has only to do with you," Solomon said.

"How so?"

"My last posting before discharge from the army was in Washington, helping General Grant prepare for an invasion of Virginia to confront General Lee. It had been a year since we met in person, so I felt sure you had no interest in me."

Rachel squeezed his hand.

"I did."

"I know that now. Anyway, just before my discharge, I was having a conversation with an infantry officer and I told him of our chance meeting at Chancellorsville. He, in turn, told me of a nurse who had just been reassigned to the Army of the Potomac who had worked closely with a British female surgeon after Gettysburg."

"A nurse? There were plenty," Rachel said.

"I sought her out. Her name was Cat."

"Oh, my God, you talked to Cat Canetti. She and I were kindred spirits."

"You had confided your feelings for me to Cat. That removed any doubts about what I needed to do. Of course, I remembered every second of our conversations in Chancellorsville," Solomon said.

"As did I."

"As soon as I returned to Boston, I researched surgical manufacturing. When I learned the Weitz Company was a leader in the industry, I wrote to Mr. Weitz, hoping only to start a joint venture that would give me reason to come to London. Much to my surprise and delight, I learned he was eager to sell."

"Why didn't you write me to tell of your arrival?"

"In my first correspondence with Weitz, I asked if he knew you."

"He does. I use his instruments."

"Weitz demanded that I not meet with you for fear of alienating Sir John. Not knowing if I'd be able to break away from the negotiations with Weitz, I thought it best not to let you know I was in London and spoil the deal. Then I met you at the College of Surgeons meeting quite by chance! Afterward, Sir John grilled me at length to learn of our connection."

"You didn't meet me at the College, you rescued me," Rachel said. "What did you tell him?"

"I lied. I told him that you merely worked on my hand and I only wanted to thank you. Nothing more. Later, Lady Weitz privately urged me not to contact you. Neither Martin nor Lady Weitz have any idea that you and the countess are friends."

"And here we are," Rachel said.

"Yes. I could have never arranged this by myself."

"You hired Robert Decker to defend me. That's not a question, because I knew it from the start. Well, that's not totally true. Do you remember Bessy? She had it figured out before me."

"I hired Robert as soon as I heard the bind you were in," Solomon said. "Our families go back a while."

"You're heading back to Boston and I don't know when I'll get to see you again. It makes me sad. There's nothing you can do about that?"

"No. My ship to Boston leaves in four days. If I could,

I would spend every second with you and not share you with the crew of *The Biscuit*. I don't want to waste a minute of our time together."

"Nor do I. I'll fix it," Rachel said.

"You'll fix it. What does that mean?"

"Trust me."

Rachel had the First Mate head for Yarmouth on the northwest tip of the Isle of Wight and drop anchor. Two seaman rowed Rachel and Solomon ashore and together they booked a room in the George Hotel as Mr. and Mrs. Birch from Boston, Massachusetts.

"Are you hungry," Solomon asked as he dropped their overnight bags in the corner of the room.

"Honestly ..." Rachel said, not answering the question but dropping her coat on a chair and undoing the draw string at the top of her blouse.

"I feel the same," Solomon said. "We can eat later."

"You read my thoughts already. I've been doing this in my mind nightly for a year. Don't move," Rachel said, as she started unbuttoning Solomon's shirt.

"We've actually spent less than an hour together before today. Are we crazy?" Solomon asked as Rachel undressed him.

"Yes. Insane, actually, but we are not crazy," Rachel said. "We met a year and a half ago and there's not been a day when I haven't thought or dreamed of you. I don't care what little time we've spent together. It's enough for me to know."

After Rachel had removed Solomon's shirt, he started to lift her blouse, but moved too quickly.

Rachel said, "You could go slower."

Solomon shook his head. "I'm too old at thirty-one to wait for anything I don't have to wait for. Like you, I've dreamt of nothing else but being with you since the night we met. It's how I got through the last year traipsing through northern Virginia with the Army of the Potomac."

"Did you worry I wouldn't wait?" Rachel asked as her blouse came off.

"Of course, I worried. Sometimes, my dreams were dark. But after meeting Cat, all doubts were erased," Solomon said, as he loosened the cinch on his pants.

"I had no doubts. You can ask my aunt and uncle. I talked about you every day."

"I did wonder that my memory of you might have been blurred by fear, pain and laudanum."

"It will do that."

"But seeing you on the podium at the College meeting," Solomon said, "standing tall and so breathtakingly beautiful, lecturing to a group of self-indulgent surgeons who were anxious to bury you, I knew. I had tears in my eyes, I was so certain I wanted to be with you any way I could."

Rachel pulled her camisole over her head and they now stood naked, facing each other.

"Have we gone too fast?" Solomon asked again. "I'll not force the issue."

Rachel giggled.

"What's so funny?" Solomon asked.

"You said it yourself," Rachel whispered. "We're both old enough not to waste even a second more of our lives. If you do not force the issue, I will."

Solomon pulled back the covers of the bed and they melted into each other, exploring each part with lips, fingers and tongues. Him gentle but firm, her submissive, until the tables turned and she wanted more and more, deeper and deeper, as she pulled herself into him until there was nothing more to give.

As they lay face to face, the only light coming from the single wick of a kerosene lantern, she asked, "Must you return to Boston?"

"You know I must," Solomon said. "I've three things to do."

"Those are?" Rachel asked, as she rolled Solomon over then moved to straddle him.

"First, convince my family we should buy an experienced surgical tool manufacturer, allowing me to return to London. Second, find a way for you to return to the United States."

"And the other?"

"Tell my family I'm getting married."

Rachel's head popped back. "Are you proposing?"

"Yes, I am."

"Then I accept," Rachel said, leaning down and kissing Solomon again. "Do I get a ring?"

"I thought I was merely going sailing," Solomon said, laughing. "I came unprepared."

"Oh, you are sailing," Rachel said. "But will the waters be smooth or not?"

Solomon's brow furrowed wryly.

"Perhaps a little choppy. Martin Weitz should sell his company as he has no workable heir. But the price he's asking, though fair, is more than my family will spend by a half. Also –" he paused, wearing an apologetic expression – "convincing my family that I should marry you won't be easy. Family meaning my mother."

"You said yourself that I'm perfect."

"Yes, I did. You're exquisitely beautiful, smart, adventurous, love boating, you're a surgeon, and Jewish. My family would adore you."

"Where's the rub?" Rachel asked.

"You're an enemy of the United States, were deported, you've purchased slaves, fought for the Confederacy, and finally, you live in England whilst I have a business to run in Boston," Solomon said. "My mother harps on the negatives every time I bring you up."

"Those can be explained," Rachel said.

"You don't know my mother. She is a force of nature and tries to dissuade me on each count. She was certain this trip would end badly."

"I pray that it will not end badly," Rachel said. "I pray it will not end."

After ordering hot water to the room to bathe, Rachel and Solomon went to a pub for a light supper then returned to the hotel. They made love again and talked until one in the morning. Six hours later they were dockside, waiting to be rowed back to *The Biscuit.*

The cruise back to Southampton went smoothly. The crew and Solomon sat with Rachel at lunch. Swearing them all to secrecy, she told the story of the Cowes Week race in detail.

Only then, from one of the crew, did she learn that Ol' Tom Voz had died a few months earlier. Rachel stood and walked away from the crew. Solomon understood her sadness and followed her to the front of the sloop where she stood silently, her arms wrapped around her chest. Solomon encircled her in his arms but knew nothing could be said.

Apparently, Ol' Tom told all those in Bournemouth who would listen that he hadn't captained the *Glory B* for the Queen's cup that day, but refused to swear to it, nor would he swear that a young woman hadn't been on the crew. He did swear to winning one-hundred-ten pounds on a ten-pound wager.

As *The Biscuit* neared the dock in Southampton, Rachel told Solomon more of her relationship to Ol' Tom Voz. "I'll be sad for today thinking of him but I know he died happy with a son and a mate. He was the best."

Back in Southampton that night, Solomon gave away his room at the yacht club and left a message for the Countess that he'd be at the Star Hotel.

The next morning, Olivia retrieved Solomon for the trip back to London. Rachel stayed back and took the next train. When she returned home that evening, she told Cynthia and Simon everything – including the nights spent with Solomon on the Isle of Wight and the Star Hotel.

"I'm too old to keep secrets from you," she said.

"Despite all the obstacles, he asked me to marry him and I said yes."

"Indeed, so many obstacles," Simon said.

Solomon did not see Rachel again and sailed back to America two days later. Rachel cried on Cynthia's shoulder the entire day.

"Will he return?" Rachel asked Cynthia, more prayer than question.

"I hope so," Cynthia said. "You deserve every happiness."

Rachel lamented the obvious. "If he and his family cannot purchase the Weitz Company and I cannot enter the United States, we are doomed."

After her presentation, Rachel thought the College would reconsider her application. She reapplied to become a Fellow of the Royal College of Surgeons. Her rejection letter arrived a week later.

Simon re-submitted their paper on hypochlorite scrubbing to six journals in England and Europe. Within six months, all six rejected the paper. Mr. Joseph Lister, the Glasgow surgeon who believed Rachel and Simon's research had merit, invited Rachel to deliver her research to the physicians of Glasgow. It received a lukewarm response.

Two months after Solomon set sail for home, Rachel received her first letter from him. She read it alone first, then out loud to Cynthia and Simon.

> *January 14,1865*
> *Dearest Rachel,*
> *I think of you every moment. Do not despair, as soon as I arrived home, I went to work solving our problems.*
>
> *I've sent an offer to Martin Weitz to purchase his company for a price our family can afford, one-hundred-thousand pounds.*

Weitz refused the offer, but countered at one-hundred-twenty-five-thousand pounds, which I believe to be a fair price and well below his company's worth. My biggest fear is that Mr. Weitz will sell to another firm before we can raise the additional capital.

As to your status as an undesirable, George Decker is friends with the Governor of Massachusetts, John Andrew. He has approached Mr. Andrew about using his influence in Washington to remove the sentence given to you and your uncle. Andrew's opinion is that the Union needs to win the war first before any approach to the Department of Justice has a chance of success.

As you know, Mr. Lincoln has just been elected President again. The Attorney General, Edward Bates, and his assistant attorney, Ted Burns, are not likely to change. Decker believes Bates and Burns thought you should have been thrown in prison. We may have to wait for a change of administrations for us to have a chance of changing your status.

Alas, my dear, your return to the States may not be possible until 1868 or later.

As to my love for you, it is as strong as ever. As to my proposal for marriage, I remain steadfast. As to our third obstacle, my mother is softening. I bombard her daily with your attributes.

Expect a delivery in the next few weeks.

Love,
Solomon

"There's nothing to do but wait, I suppose," Simon said.

"You poor darling," Cynthia said. "Waiting is not your strong suit. I hope he doesn't find another."

"He'll wait. That much I'm sure of," Rachel said.

The following day, Rachel, not one to sit idly by, went to the Bank of London to check on her finances. After her costly escapade in America, her bankers told her she could afford to invest twelve-thousand-five-hundred pounds, but not a penny more.

She asked Simon if he would invest in Solomon's venture. The response from Simon and Cynthia was an immediate 'NO!'

Cynthia, almost in tears, said, "We've had too many friends lose everything by investing in schemes in which they had no control."

Simon added, "You'd be a minority party without a leg to stand on. You could easily lose every farthing, whilst the majority holders secret away whatever they can find. I won't hear of it."

"I trust Solomon," Rachel insisted.

Cynthia and Simon could only shake their heads.

That same day, Rachel received a note from Olivia, summoning her to Brown's Hotel in two days' time.

Rachel curtsied as she approached the table.

Olivia laughed. "You needn't curtsy at a restaurant. Besides, it draws attention to me, which I don't need."

"How will I know which is an official meeting and which is not," Rachel said, sitting. "Besides, I enjoy doing it for you."

"No one enjoys curtsying whom I know of," Olivia said with head shake. "I don't enjoy it when I visit the royals."

"I enjoy doing it for you."

"You've said you're an odd duck. I'd have to agree with your self-assessment," Olivia chuckled. "The First Mate on *The Biscuit* told me you entertained the crew at every opportunity and went further with Solomon than I would have guessed."

"You're not going to ask me if I offered sexual favors, are you?" Rachel asked, with a smile.

"I've made that mistake once. I won't again," Olivia responded. "So tell me of your time with him."

"He proposed marriage the first night," Rachel said. "I accepted."

"I see no ring."

"He thought he was only going boating with you. He didn't think an engagement ring was needed."

Olivia laughed again. "True. I've seen Lady Weitz a few times since. She still suspects nothing of our gambit."

"I still have unsolvable issues, unfortunately."

"Tell me. I love issues," Olivia said.

"I'm considered an enemy of the United States for starters," Rachel said. "His mother is a tough nut, but he writes that she's softening. Lastly, he wants to buy Martin Weitz's business but needs a bit more capital."

"I can do nothing about the mother," Olivia said. "I'll think on you being an enemy of our colonies. But I'd like to know more about Weitz's offering. Martin Weitz is held in high regard for his business acumen and the quality of his instruments, but Linda tells me he's tired and would like to sell. His son-in-law is a ne'er-do-well and both sons want only to be gentlemen and court women with sordid pasts."

"That's what Solomon surmised," Rachel said. "Weitz has no debt and offered the company at well below its market value: one-hundred-twenty-five thousand pounds. The number is still a bit above Solomon's ability to pay by a quarter. Solomon is afraid someone will scoop it up before he can raise the additional funds. For what it's worth, I use Weitz's instruments exclusively at St. James."

"How much more does he need?" Olivia asked.

"Solomon doesn't know I'm trying to raise the

difference. He needs twenty-five thousand pounds. My bankers tell me they won't let me use more than half of that for a one-tenth share."

"Your bankers?" Olivia asked, startled. "I would have assumed you were getting money from your uncle."

"My aunt and uncle want no part of this."

"How then did you amass that much money?" Olivia inquired. "Certainly not at St. James Charity. I know they pay you close to nothing?"

"My father was quite wealthy and left me his entire estate," Rachel said.

"Did Andrew know this?" Olivia asked, looking flabbergasted.

"Thinking us poor, Andrew said he'd figure out some way to make ends meet without staying in the army. He was going to read law with your husband's cousin. Only then did I tell him of my endowment."

"I admit," Olivia said, "you have amazing surprises to present every time we meet. Like a magician who keeps pulling rabbit after rabbit out of a top hat."

"I hope that's good," Rachel said.

"Might I make the difference?" Olivia asked. "I love the earl dearly, but he says women have no business sense. I'd like to show my daughter and two sons that we do."

"I had no intention of asking you," Rachel said.

"I know."

"Are you serious?"

"Absolutely. I'd like nothing more than to be partners with you and own a piece of Weitz's company," Olivia said.

Their lunch lasted another hour. Rachel rushed to the London office of the Atlantic Telegraph Company and paid twenty pounds to send a telegram to Boston via Newfoundland, Canada.

August 21, 1865
Solomon Birch

12 Market Street
Lowell, Massachusetts
I have secured twenty-five thousand pounds.
Buy it.
Rachel

Chapter Twenty-one
Weitz

Rachel received a telegram from Solomon two days later, saying that he'd be back in London in two weeks.

The next day, Rachel received a package containing a two-carat diamond engagement ring from R. Phillips Goldsworthy jewelers.

Rachel met Solomon dockside in Liverpool. Together they took the train to London.

"We mustn't let Weitz know the source of the additional funds," Solomon said. "Sir John still advises him and appears at every meeting we had on my first visit."

"I figured as much," Rachel said. "I've booked you a room at the Clermont Hotel. But you must meet with my aunt and uncle, and then the supplier of the rest of the money."

"Who might that be?" Solomon asked. "I have no idea where the money is coming from."

"Half and half, me and Olivia, the Countess," Rachel said.

"You?" Solomon asked in confusion. "Do you mean your uncle?"

"He wanted no part of it," Rachel said. "My father's estate made me a rich woman. I've never used it other than to fund my escapade to the States."

"I had no idea," Solomon said.

"We're both eager to own a tenth share of this enterprise. We understand the percentage will be diminished if Weitz is melded into your company in Boston."

"We'll keep it separate in the beginning, per my family's wishes," Solomon said.

Solomon met with Simon and Cynthia the next morning at their home. Knowing their marriage was now a foregone conclusion, Simon and Cynthia had decided to like Solomon no matter how he presented. Fortuitously, they fell in love with Solomon in an instant.

"Where will you reside when you take the reins at Weitz?" Simon asked.

Without hesitation, Rachel answered, "He's agreed to live here with us whilst in London."

"I did?" Solomon asked.

"Yes. You didn't know it 'til now," Rachel said, smiling. "This house is big enough for another four couples."

Solomon and Rachel then met with Olivia at the Bank of London office. Olivia had her lawyers draw up an agreement so that she and Rachel were silent partners in the Martin Weitz Company with a one-tenth share each.

The next day, Solomon met with Martin Weitz and Sir John Minkove and purchased Weitz's company. Solomon had already demanded he retain the name The Weitz Company. Martin Weitz and Sir John would remain as consultants for the next two years with a salary of five hundred pounds per year.

Until the completion of the sale, neither Weitz nor Sir John knew that Rachel and Olivia were silent partners. Solomon and Rachel agreed that she would need time to smooth the waters with Sir John before the truth came out.

At dinner that night at Simon and Cynthia's home with Olivia as a guest, Solomon talked of the remaining two problems to their marriage: his mother and Rachel's status with the Department of Justice.

"Lee is being chased all over Virginia by Grant," Solomon said. "His men are starving and the South is out of troops and supplies. The Union has control of the west and the Mississippi River while Sherman marches through Georgia putting flames to everything. It will be over soon."

"Will I then be able to meet your family?" Rachel

asked.

"It is possible, but not guaranteed. Once the war is over, many of the Southern inciters will be put to trial for the rebellion," Solomon said. "Lincoln is sympathetic, however, so I'm hopeful that not too much retribution will be exacted."

"There's another problem that I have," Cynthia said. "Neighbors and friends." She looked at Solomon. You two are unmarried and sharing a bedroom. People talk, ask questions, and I have to answer them or they assume the worst."

"We understood this would happen. We've the solution but haven't told you," Solomon said.

"And that is?" Cynthia asked.

"On Monday morning, we shall be married in a civil ceremony with all of you as witnesses."

"Just like that?" Cynthia said.

"Yes, but I'd like to keep it secret from my family. I want us to be married by our rabbi in Boston," Solomon said. "Our family is huge and it would mean the world to my mother to have the ceremony at home."

"Oh," Cynthia said. "I had hoped we might do it here."

After an uncomfortable silence, Olivia asked, "Solomon, do you travel north to Canada often?"

"My mother's younger sister, Joyce, married a Montreal snake-oil merchant named Marcel Nemirow. He's done all right though as a member of the shoddyocracy.[36] Joyce turns sixty in September and the family is going north to celebrate. Why?"

"First, can you not speak the Queen's English?" Olivia asked. "What in God's name is 'shoddyocracy'?"

---

[36] Shoddyocracy: 1800s American slang term referring to a group of people who become wealthy by selling low-quality merchandise.

Chapter Twenty-two
Montreal

Solomon stayed in London for three months. Craftsmen and salespeople from the Birch Company in Lowell, Massachusetts, came to London to learn the techniques required to manufacture, service and sell surgical equipment in the American market. Rachel and Simon made peace with Sir John Minkove and together they helped in the transition. Solomon headed home at the end of August and would not divulge his marriage to Rachel.

As planned, the Birch family headed north to Montreal on the first weekend of September for Aunt Joyce's sixtieth birthday. Solomon had told his mother he would sail afterward from Montreal to England to complete the takeover and running of The Weitz Company. Little did the Birch family know that Cynthia had arrived in Montreal in mid-August in time to work with Aunt Joyce to plan the birthday and a surprise wedding.

That Cynthia spoke French fluently, while Joyce did not, made things easier. Even the rabbi from Solomon's Boston congregation secretly agreed to come north for the festivities. As Canada remained a British Protectorate, Rachel had no difficulty entering a week before the wedding.

The party was held in the small ballroom of the Donegan Hotel. A chuppah, or wedding canopy, was erected in the middle of the ballroom. As the Boston family arrived, Aunt Joyce, Rachel, the Birch family rabbi, Cynthia, and Simon stood together next to the chuppah. The new arrivals scratched their heads at presence of their rabbi and a chuppah in the middle of a supposed birthday bash.

Upon entry, Solomon's mother, Edith Birch, scanned the room and walked immediately to her sister. Solomon, knowing the plot, followed his mother. After the obligatory hug and kiss, Edith said, "I'm missing something. You're happily married and so are your two children. What's our rabbi doing here with a chuppah?"

Edith looked to the right, at a smiling Rachel. "And who's this young lady dressed in a wedding gown?"

Suddenly, the truth hit Edith and she turned back to her sister. "Oh my God. Don't tell me." Edith turned to Solomon, who had taken Rachel's hand, and then back to her sister, Joyce. "You sneak. I didn't know."

"Oh, you haven't met?" Joyce laughed. "My dear sister Edith, this is Dr. Rachel Romain, a surgeon from London, who, by the end of the evening, will be your daughter-in-law. Behind Rachel are her aunt and uncle, Cynthia and Simon Romain."

"You planned all this without telling me?" Edith whined. "How could you?"

"Solomon pleaded with me to work with Rachel's Aunt Cynthia who came three weeks ago," Joyce said. "I thought it a grand idea. The family was coming anyway."

Joyce leaned into Edith and whispered, "The Romains are footing the bill. How could I refuse."

Edith, shaking her head, had to sit to collect her thoughts. Rachel and Solomon sat next to her.

Edith turned to Solomon and said, "Go away for a bit. I'm mad because you've deprived me of planning a wedding."

Solomon shrugged and walked away.

Edith faced Rachel. "So, you are real? All Solomon talks about when he's home is Rachel, Rachel, Rachel. You're quite a remarkable woman. I expected you to fly into the room with wings of gold and a crown of diamonds and rubies."

"Sorry to disappoint. It's only ordinary me," Rachel said.

"Ordinary, never. If only half the things Solomon has told me are true." Edith then stood and said, "What a wonderful surprise. Stand and give me a hug, then I'll introduce you to the family."

As Rachel and Edith hugged, Robert Decker, Catherine 'Cat' Canetti, Bessy and Flora entered the room to surprise Rachel.

Epilogue

Simon, Cynthia, Solomon and Rachel headed back to London after the wedding. As expected, Cynthia swore she would never step foot on a ship again. Rachel returned to St. James Charity as Solomon took over management of the Martin Weitz Company, traveling back to Boston every three months.

Rachel continued to practice until her seventh month of pregnancy. On May 1st, 1866, she delivered healthy twins: a boy, Jacob, and a girl, Gayle. Two years later, another boy, Paul, was born.

The Weitz Company had been the leading British manufacturer of surgical equipment. Within two years, it became the leader in the United States as well.

Olivia and Rachel earned twenty thousand pounds each in the first year for their twelve-thousand-five-hundred-pound investment. Each year the earnings increased until Olivia earned more yearly than her husband, the Earl.

Each year, Rachel applied for membership in the Royal College of Surgeons. Each year her application was denied.

Even more frustrating for Edith, Solomon and Rachel were their attempts to gain Rachel access to the United States. It wasn't until 1877 when Rutherford B. Hayes became the nineteenth president and installed Charles Devens as Attorney General. Devens had been a Civil War hero, wounded three times, and a general who distinguished himself at Chancellorsville, Cold Harbor, and the Siege of Petersburg. After the war, Devens returned to his home state of Massachusetts and became a Massachusetts Supreme Court Justice. Robert Decker had presented multiple times in front of Devens and approached him, as a friend, to see about lifting the restriction on Rachel coming to the United States.

In July, 1879, Solomon, Rachel and their three children stepped off an ocean liner in Boston to visit the

Birch family. For the next fifteen years, Solomon and Rachel would spend each July yachting at the Birch summer home on Cape Cod.

Cynthia and Simon Romain died five months apart in 1885. In 1886, Sir John Minkove, in his eighties and long since retired, delivered an address to the Fellows apologizing for not accepting Rachel and Simon's work, now proven to be accurate based on Joseph Lister's work[37]. The only dissenter to Rachel's work was Robert Kennedy, Jr. from Belfast, who still didn't believe in sterile surgical technique or vaccinations for smallpox.

When Kennedy raised objections after Minkove's address, Minkove responded to Kennedy by saying, "Robert, you can't teach stupidity."

Rachel and Solomon would continue to reside in the

---

[37] *Mr. Joseph Lister of Glasgow continued to work on the answer to wound putrefaction and infection. At the Glasgow Royal Infirmary as late as 1865, the death rate for amputations in Lister's wards remained above thirty percent. Lister's father, Joseph Jackson Lister, was a famous microscopist, a member of the Royal Society, and he taught his son to use the microscope.*

In 1865, Joseph Lister learned of Louis Pasteur's work on alcohol fermentation and infection caused by microorganisms. Lister accepted Pasteur's theories as they pertained to wound infection. He also found that the use of carbolic acid, a chemical used to clean sewers, was less toxic for human use than chlorine or bromine solutions. When Lister started using carbolic acid to clean instruments and hands, his infection rate fell dramatically. From this, Lister published his seminal work, On a New Method of treating Compound Fracture, Abscess, Etc., with Observations on the Conditions of Suppuration and On the Antiseptic Principle in the Practice of Surgery.

Lister traveled across Europe and the United States preaching of his discoveries. Like many innovations, acceptance of germ theory met strong resistance, especially in the United States. Most notable was the unsterile probing used by surgeons in treating James Garfield, Twentieth President of the United States, in 1881. Garfield died from iatrogenic[37] infection ten weeks after an assassination attempt. By 1890, Lister's theories were finally accepted worldwide.

Romain home for the rest of their lives.

Rachel retired from surgery at the age of sixty-five, never having been accepted into the Royal College of Surgeons. She died in 1902, at the age of sixty-eight. Solomon died two years later while visiting Cape Cod.

Rachel and Olivia remained close friends their entire lives and met the first Wednesday of every month for lunch at Brown's Hotel. Olivia was godmother to all three of Rachel's children. As promised, Rachel and her family received invitations to the Earl and Countess's Christmas dinner every year.

Solomon and Rachel's son, Paul, became a barrister in the English legal system. Though quite successful, he resigned his position and went to work for the Royal Merchant Navy as a lobbyist.

Gayle, their daughter, married a surgeon and worked as a surgical nurse for a while, but retired to raise children. She became an avid golfer, finishing second in the inaugural Wimbledon Lady's Golf tourney in 1893. Her husband refused to play golf, not wishing to be thrashed by his wife.

Jacob became a surgeon and a Fellow in the Royal College of Surgeons. He pleaded yearly to have his mother be accepted into the College even after her death.

Finally, in 1912, the Royal College of Surgeons inducted Dr. Rachel Romain, posthumously, as a Fellow, a year after Miss Eleanor Davies-Colley became the first female Fellow of the Royal College of Surgeons.

As a Fellow, and following the Royal College of Surgeon's tradition of dropping 'Doctor' from her name, Dr. Rachel Romain became Mrs. Rachel Birch, FRCS.

ABOUT THE AUTHOR

James Gottesman, M.D. is a Urological Oncologist who has been writing for most of his adult life. He graduated from UC Berkeley and UC San Francisco Medical Center and did his urology residency at UCLA; he has authored more than 100 scientific papers, medical book chapters, research grants, and medically unique computer programs. He was Clinical Professor of Urology at the University of Washington and Chief of Urology at Swedish Medical Center in Seattle.

Dr. Gottesman's previous books of fiction include *The Road Back Isn't Straight* (2013), *The Search of Grace* (2014), *Can't Forget* (2016), *Stab Wound* (2019), *An Enemy to Love* (2021), *In Flew Enza* (2022), and *The Angel of North Africa* (2024). He lives on Mercer Island, Washington, with his wife Gloria and their dog, Biscuit, near their three sons and nine grandchildren.

Made in the USA
Middletown, DE
16 February 2026

28157528R00166